国家出版基金项目
NATIONAL PUBLICATION FOUNDATION

纳米科学与技术

生产与工作场所纳米颗粒暴露监测指南

陈春英 陈 瑞 白 茹 赵宇亮 编著

科学出版社

北 京

内 容 简 介

纳米颗粒暴露现场的安全问题,是纳米科技走向产业化必须面临的核心问题,也是科技发达国家在可持续发展战略中,最为重视和优先考虑的问题。

我国正处在从纳米科技大国向纳米科技强国转化的关键时机,纳米技术相关产业的发展,是衡量这个转化过程是否成功的关键。为了支撑这个转化过程,我们在过去十余年的研究工作基础上,结合国际上的相关进展,在本书中针对生产场所以及工作场所中纳米颗粒的暴露监测以及相关安全性所涉及的各个方面,进行了系统全面的论述。首先,综述了生产场所以及工作场所中纳米颗粒暴露的相关知识,包括现场环境中颗粒物的表征方法、典型纳米材料生产现场的颗粒物暴露国内外重要研究进展等。其次,对暴露现场监测中的具体策略、技术方法和仪器设备进行了详细的阐述。最后,针对纳米颗粒暴露现场的风险评价和安全防护,根据已有的研究结果给出了不同纳米材料的空气暴露剂量阈值(建议值),提出了指导建议与操作方法。此外,本书附录部分还提供了近年来国内在纳米安全前沿领域产出的重要研究成果摘要。

本书可为相关专业的研究生与本科生、纳米科技领域的科研人员、气溶胶科学领域的研究人员、预防与劳动卫生工作者等提供参考,尤其是为我国纳米生产相关企业、政府监督管理部门在制定相关政策法规、建立纳米产业安全措施与防护方法上提供科学依据。

图书在版编目(CIP)数据

生产与工作场所纳米颗粒暴露监测指南/陈春英等编著. —北京:科学出版社,2015.9
(纳米科学与技术/白春礼主编)
ISBN 978-7-03-045860-5

Ⅰ.①生… Ⅱ.①陈… Ⅲ.①纳米材料-超微粒子-有害物质-环境监测-指南 Ⅳ.①X83-62②R134-62

中国版本图书馆 CIP 数据核字(2015)第 226642 号

责任编辑:杨 震 刘 冉 / 责任校对:郑金红
责任印制:徐晓晨 / 封面设计:陈 敬

科学出版社 出版
北京东黄城根北街 16 号
邮政编码:100717
http://www.sciencep.com

北京凌奇印刷有限责任公司 印刷
科学出版社发行 各地新华书店经销

*

2015 年 9 月第 一 版 开本:720×1000 1/16
2019 年 4 月第三次印刷 印张:12 3/4
字数:260 000

定价:80.00 元
(如有印装质量问题,我社负责调换)

《纳米科学与技术》丛书序

在新兴前沿领域的快速发展过程中,及时整理、归纳、出版前沿科学的系统性专著,一直是发达国家在国家层面上推动科学与技术发展的重要手段,是一个国家保持科学技术的领先权和引领作用的重要策略之一。

科学技术的发展和应用,离不开知识的传播:我们从事科学研究,得到了"数据"(论文),这只是"信息"。将相关的大量信息进行整理、分析,使之形成体系并付诸实践,才变成"知识"。信息和知识如果不能交流,就没有用处,所以需要"传播"(出版),这样才能被更多的人"应用",被更有效地应用,被更准确地应用,知识才能产生更大的社会效益,国家才能在越来越高的水平上发展。所以,数据→信息→知识→传播→应用→效益→发展,这是科学技术推动社会发展的基本流程。其中,知识的传播,无疑具有桥梁的作用。

整个 20 世纪,我国在及时地编辑、归纳、出版各个领域的科学技术前沿的系列专著方面,已经大大地落后于科技发达国家,其中的原因有许多,我认为更主要的是缘于科学文化的习惯不同:中国科学家不习惯去花时间整理和梳理自己所从事的研究领域的知识,将其变成具有系统性的知识结构。所以,很多学科领域的第一本原创性"教科书",大都来自欧美国家。当然,真正优秀的著作不仅需要花费时间和精力,更重要的是要有自己的学术思想以及对这个学科领域充分把握和高度概括的学术能力。

纳米科技已经成为 21 世纪前沿科学技术的代表领域之一,其对经济和社会发展所产生的潜在影响,已经成为全球关注的焦点。国际纯粹与应用化学联合会(IUPAC)会刊在 2006 年 12 月评论:"现在的发达国家如果不发展纳米科技,今后必将沦为第三世界发展中国家。"因此,世界各国,尤其是科技强国,都将发展纳米科技作为国家战略。

兴起于 20 世纪后期的纳米科技,给我国提供了与科技发达国家同步发展的良好机遇。目前,各国政府都在加大力度出版纳米科技领域的教材、专著以及科普读物。在我国,纳米科技领域尚没有一套能够系统、科学地展现纳米科学技术各个方面前沿进展的系统性专著。因此,国家纳米科学中心与科学出版社共同发起并组织出版《纳米科学与技术》,力求体现本领域出版读物的科学性、准确性和系统性,全面科学地阐述纳米科学技术前沿、基础和应用。本套丛书的出版以高质量、科学性、准确性、系统性、实用性为目标,将涵盖纳米科学技术的所有领域,全面介绍国内外纳米科学技术发展的前沿知识;并长期组织专家撰写、编辑出版下去,为我国纳米科技各个相关基础学科和技术领域的科技工作者和研究生、本科生等,提供一套重要的参考资料。

这是我们努力实践"科学发展观"思想的一次创新,也是一件利国利民、对国家科学技术发展具有重要意义的大事。感谢科学出版社给我们提供的这个平台,这不仅有助于我国在科研一线工作的高水平科学家逐渐增强归纳、整理和传播知识的主动性(这也是科学研究回馈和服务社会的重要内涵之一),而且有助于培养我国各个领域的人士对前沿科学技术发展的敏感性和兴趣爱好,从而为提高全民科学素养作出贡献。

我谨代表《纳米科学与技术》编委会,感谢为此付出辛勤劳动的作者、编委会委员和出版社的同仁们。

同时希望您,尊贵的读者,如获此书,开卷有益!

中国科学院院长
国家纳米科技指导协调委员会首席科学家
2011 年 3 月于北京

前　　言

　　纳米科学技术是步入 21 世纪以来，一直受到人们广泛追捧的科技"宠儿"。纳米是一种几何尺寸的度量单位，1 纳米＝百万分之一毫米。纳米技术是一门交叉性很强的综合学科，研究的内容涉及现代科技的广阔领域。与物理学、化学、材料学、生物学、电子学、力学等学科相互渗透，其中纳米材料的制备和研究是整个纳米科技的基础。在一定条件下，颗粒物质会随着尺寸的变小，能引起宏观物理性质上的变化，这被称作小尺寸效应，同时，纳米颗粒本身能够产生一系列新奇的性质上的变化，这些特有的性质可用于科技发展的方方面面。随着纳米科技的迅猛发展，各种人造纳米材料已经在医药、化妆品和电子等产品中广泛使用，而以商业性为目的纳米相关材料的工业化生产与加工规模在逐渐增大，也已经越来越广泛。任何事物的出现与发展都有其两面性，纳米科技也不例外。那么随着纳米科技发展会带来哪些安全性上的问题呢？

　　总体来说，纳米科技还没有完全成熟，未来的发展与成熟还具有很大的不确定性。与纳米相关原材料及产品生产和加工现场颗粒物释放与暴露，已成为国内外政府部门以及企业管理人员高度关注的问题。与生产和实验室制备等直接相关的是处于工作一线的广大劳动人员，他们处于纳米科技的前线，属于最容易产生高暴露风险的人群。如果能够特异性降低此特定人群的风险概率，则可以从纳米科技全局上，大大增加纳米科技安全性系数，降低人们极端情况下的风险暴露概率，避免产生由现场暴露引发的健康危害及其对纳米科技可持续发展的损害。

　　其实，大气可吸入颗粒物污染本身就包括纳米级颗粒物的污染问题，并日益引起各国的高度重视。大气环境科学研究已侧重于针对 $PM_{2.5}$（$\leqslant 2.5$ μm）甚至超细颗粒物（纳米）对环境的危害研究，同时，人们早已意识到大气超细颗粒物污染与心血管疾病之间的重要联系。类似于大气污染，不同工业生产现场存在不同程度的气溶胶污染，众多工作环境内存在粉尘或纳米级颗粒物的污染，如广为人知的吸入金属加工过程中的金属烟雾，能使工人患帕金森症的概率大大高于普通人；诸如煤矿、钛白粉厂、矿石厂和石棉相关企业由长时间吸入粉尘而造成的矽肺、肺气肿或肺癌等肺病早已为人所熟知。另外，2014 年 8 月发生的昆山中荣金属制品有限公司抛光二车间特别重大铝粉尘爆炸事故，从现场颗粒释放暴露影响健康的问题直接上升到了重大生产责任事故，令人痛心。这与企业对粉尘颗粒的控制缺乏必要监测,没有及时清理工艺设备或通风系统中的粉尘,金属粉尘悬浮于空中聚集到一定程度时,达到爆炸浓度极限密切相关。纳米生产相关现场可能存在类似的问题,由于纳米颗粒的特殊性,不仅需要考虑呼吸暴露,同时需要考虑通过其他路径产生的暴露方式,比如皮肤污染。在某些实例中,已经发现不能明显区分纳米颗粒与其他污染物造成的暴露以及潜在的健康危害,如果不能正确地表征纳米颗粒物的释放与暴露情况,则很容易造成错误的结论。评价方法的空白使人们很容易把其他因素引起的综合效应,一概归咎于纳米颗粒。因此,针对纳米生产与工作现场颗粒暴露情况的研究工作,可以正确地评估纳米颗粒的释放和空气动力学行为,为建立合理的职业防护方案提供技术指导,为建立纳米颗粒职业暴露阈值提供重要依据。使纳米科技更贴近实际,不至于重走新兴技术出现就易被"妖魔化"的老套道路。

目前,针对纳米生产场所以及现场安全生产和职业防护的相关管理规范、政策或指南在国内几乎是空白。基于这种现实情况,本书从社会实际需求与科学技术发展的角度,根据自己的研究成果,综合了世界范围内特别是欧盟、美国与日本的经验总结,编著形成了《生产与工作场所纳米颗粒暴露监测指南》一书。本书定位于基础与应用相结合,总体分为七章,主要涵盖以下内容,首先综述了纳米颗粒现场暴露的相关知识,探讨现场监测的必要性,包括现场颗粒的具体表征方法总结,同时对已有典型纳米颗粒的现场研究成果进展进行分类总结;其次,对暴露现场监测中的具体策略、方法和仪器进行了尤为详尽的阐述,涵盖具体策略、现场监测实施步骤及监测结果录入表格信息等,以期让现场监测人员能够在实际工作中灵活运用,获得生产与工作场所纳米颗粒的环境释放与团聚行为的动态变化规律,为后续建立相应的职业防护和职业风险评估提供基础数据。最后,本书针对纳米颗粒暴露现场的风险评估和安全防护,给出了具体的指导建议与操作方法。此外,本书汇聚了近年来我国在纳米安全领域所做出的创新成果,这些成果为纳米颗粒暴露的现场安全研究提供必要的毒理学与安全性评价的知识,纳米安全的知识体系是建立科学客观评价纳米产品安全性的基石。

在全球化发展的今天,高科技的健康稳定发展代表了一个国家、一个民族的希望,而高科技发展过程中可能遇到的某些问题不是一国一己所能解决的。作为纳米科技从业人员,自身能力与知识都是有限的,我们希望能在纳米颗粒暴露现场监测与评估方面抛砖引玉,与国内外同行一道,建立相应的理论与规范,为纳米科技的发展保驾护航。

本书由国家纳米科学中心陈春英、陈瑞、白茹、赵宇亮等研究人员共同起草编写,总结了我们过去十余年的研究成果,吸取了国际上的重要研究进展,汇聚了科研人员多年来的工作与思考。近几年来,作者的研究工作得到了科技部重大研究计划、国家自然科学基金、中国科学院和欧盟第七框架纳米安全研究项目的支持，得到了国内众多专家学者的指教和帮助，在此一并表示感谢。在本书即将出版之际，对参与本书编写和整理以及相关生产现场工作的所有老师和同学表示衷心的谢意！感谢在书稿的编辑和出版过程中付出辛苦努力的杨震编辑和刘冉编辑。

　　由于纳米生产场所以及纳米相关工作场所的现场监测及安全性评价与风险评估在国内外都尚处于起步阶段，新的研究结果与知识理念不断涌现，同时也限于作者的学术水平，书中难免有遗漏、偏颇甚至错误之处，敬请读者批评指正。

作　者

2015 年 9 月

目　　录

第1章 总　　述

　　纳米材料(Nanomaterials)因其诸多优异的性能而被广泛应用于微电子、化工、环境、能源、国家安全及生物医学领域。纳米科技正处于飞速发展的阶段,但与此同时,随着纳米材料及其相关产品的大量生产以及在人们生产生活中日渐广泛的应用,使得纳米材料从生产过程到形成产品都有可能进入人们的生活,再经过废弃处理进入环境,在这一完整的生命周期(Life Cycle)内都存在产生职业暴露和人群暴露的风险概率,其可能产生的潜在健康风险日益受到广泛重视。美国国家科技委员会下属的纳米科技委员会(National Science and Technology Council, Committee on Technology, Subcommittee on Nanoscale Science, Engineering, and Technology)于 2011 年 10 月颁布了针对纳米安全领域的美国国家纳米技术计划——环境、健康与安全研究战略,从国家科技战略的角度重视纳米安全研究领域的发展[1]。欧盟劳动卫生与保护机构(European Agency for Safety and Health at Work)曾在物理、化学、生物及社会心理领域中,遴选了十大潜在影响劳动保护的危害因素,其中三项分别是:①纳米颗粒物和超细颗粒物;②柴油机尾气;③人造矿物纤维,这三项本质上具有相似性,即都属于难溶性颗粒或纤维。其遴选的理由是基于现有的资料得出的普遍结论,纳米材料相关的颗粒物和超细颗粒物具有潜在的健康危害[2]。

　　通常情况下,纳米材料在正常使用时,因不产生暴露也就不会引起健康风险,如纳米材料形成复合材料加工成计算机电路板,正常使用电路板时并不会产生纳米材料导致的相应危害。然而,对于各个不同的生产制造环节,这些纳米材料的大批量生产过程,以及含有纳米材料的复合物被加工的过程,如铣削、加工、打磨及研磨等工序,都存在纳米材料对工人潜在的释放暴露风险。为了阐明纳米颗粒的暴露风险并对其进行评估,需要制定规范性的暴露评估流程与方案,从而指导如何实施暴露监测,需要测定哪些数据,需要备案哪些材料,如何分析测量结果以及如何进行结果评估。这些问题的解答与规范性操作可以增强测量间的可重复性(同一地点不同时间的监测),或不同地点测量间数据的可比性,同时增强监测结果的有效性和结论的说服力。

　　本指南综述了针对纳米材料生产加工过程中进行暴露监测的相关事项,包括已有方案,纳米颗粒暴露方式与暴露事件,现场相关监测流程及相关防护研究。首先对在阅读本指南时可能遇到的一些共性问题,进行阐释。

1.1　什么是纳米颗粒/纳米材料?

纳米颗粒通常是指至少一个尺度处于纳米级大小的颗粒,根据 ISO /TR 27628 定义,纳米颗粒是直径(可以从几何学、空气动力学、迁移率、投影面积其至其他方法计算得到)小于 100 nm 的颗粒。这些颗粒的来源可能是自然产生,如火山灰、海风等;也可能是人类生产生活产生,比如纳米材料产品、香烟燃烧、柴油机尾气、切割和焊接产生的烟雾及燃烧等。人造纳米颗粒(Engineered Nanoparticles)是指人为加工或设计获得的具有独特性状的纳米颗粒。纳米材料是泛指外部尺寸或内部结构在纳米级大小的材料,不同于非纳米级的同类物质,纳米材料/纳米粒子具有特有的性状和特征,例如金属或金属氧化物、炭黑、碳纳米管、富勒烯、硅酸盐、有机纳米颗粒或纳米复合材料等。纳米颗粒通常是指单独的颗粒,而不涉及其聚合或团聚后的存在形式,而在现实中,通常将纳米颗粒团聚后的存在状态作为纳米物质,所以纳米颗粒包含了团聚或聚合后存在的情况。

通常情况下,纳米颗粒的暴露途径分为呼吸道吸入、皮肤接触或者消化道摄入,而通过呼吸进入人体是工作场所最为可能的暴露方式。流行病学研究发现超细颗粒物可以引起肺部疾病、免疫系统及心血管系统损伤,所以,呼吸暴露是当前的研究热点。

纳米颗粒暴露主要分为职业暴露、消费品暴露及环境暴露。其中,职业暴露是纳米颗粒暴露中剂量最高、危险系数最大的环节,例如气相合成或者在粉末状材料运输包装等工作过程。当然,在清洁和维护过程或者纳米材料生命周期中的其他阶段也可能造成人体暴露,比如使用油漆、涂料时的喷雾操作,切割或锯铣纳米复合材料过程,以及材料废弃、丢弃过程。

通常如二氧化钛或者炭黑等材料都是工业化生产,这些材料产生纳米气溶胶后的成分及性质都相对比较均一,而很多情况下现场有多种材料的合成,所以环境气溶胶中的颗粒成分复杂且变化很大。在研究纳米材料的环境暴露时,需要同时考虑不同来源的纳米颗粒成分,例如、柴油机车尾气、交通、加热设备、高温装置,其至环境中其他非纳米颗粒产生源,如沙尘等。

1.2　为什么要进行暴露评价?

为了使纳米科技能够得到广泛认可,需要对可能产生的释放、暴露情况进行风险评估,相关暴露风险及预防控制知识对于风险评估和管理极其重要,当然,没有暴露就不会有风险。暴露评价通常是基于多个原因开展,首先,揭示暴露产生的释放源并对释放过程进行表征;其次,评估防护措施的有效性;第三,检测是否符合相关职业防护暴露阈值或者自定的参考标准;暴露评价也可用于建立释放暴露研究模型。总之,暴露评价的目的决定了评价过程中所采取的程序、实施过程及后续结果的判定。

1.3 何谓潜在的风险?

纳米材料相对于大尺寸材料具有很多不同的特性,一些研究表明,纳米颗粒/材料比微米大小的材料对健康具有更大的危害,这些危害可能存在于纳米材料整个生命周期的不同阶段,比如工人可能在生产、运输、储存或废弃处理阶段受到暴露;消费者可能在使用过程中暴露于纳米材料;纳米材料可通过释放进入环境,如工作环境、家庭、室外等;另外,进入外界环境的纳米材料可能会对土壤、水源、空气及动植物产生影响,环境污染同样可影响人体健康。纳米科技是一场影响社会与经济的科技革命,新技术可以解决问题,同样也可能产生新的潜在风险,形成负面的社会认知。科学家与社会学家应该鼎力合作,共同正确处理纳米材料风险暴露问题。

总之,纳米科技的发展既存在机遇,同时又迎接新的挑战。纳米颗粒现场释放暴露评估是纳米安全研究的前沿领域,必须从负责任的角度做好相关研究工作,建立科学评估规范和防护方法,为纳米安全性研究提供理性指导,从而真正让纳米科技服务国家,造福人类,这也是我们科学工作者的社会责任。

第 2 章 暴露现场纳米颗粒表征

2.1 纳米颗粒表征

2.1.1 概述

从基础研究到应用研究,从产品的生产、加工到商业化,纳米颗粒的物理化学性质表征都起着重要作用,也面临巨大挑战,例如,当气溶胶中混有纤维状颗粒时,就不能简单使用适于球形颗粒表征的仪器进行相关表征。此外,化学成分相近的纳米颗粒也可能导致截然不同的健康效应。与其他化学物质类似,纳米颗粒的物理化学性质是研究其安全性的重要参数,需详细阐明。从实验研究到安全性评价,以及制定的安全性评估方法,最终是为了降低纳米颗粒暴露风险,保护环境安全和人类健康。

已有研究表明,与宏观尺度的材料相比,具有相同化学组分的纳米材料拥有不同的理化特性,这与纳米颗粒的尺寸、形状和表面特性有关。因此,需要对纳米颗粒进行详细的物理化学性质表征,这也是研究纳米颗粒安全性的前提条件。对于使用不同制备方法得到的相同纳米材料,更加需要详细的表征以阐明不同方法以及引起的生物效应之间的差异,例如碳纳米管(Carbon Nanotubes),可以通过多种方法制备,且形状差异很大,引起的毒理学效应也不同[3,4]。Zuin 等强调,对碳纳米管、富勒醇、金属氧化物(如二氧化钛、氧化铁)、二氧化硅、量子点(Quantum Dot)等纳米材料的毒性研究,需要对其理化性质进行详细表征,然后再研究其产生的生物效应[5]。在理想情况下,纳米材料的生物效应研究应当以详细的理化性质数据为基础。

2.1.2 纳米颗粒表征面临的挑战

1. 纳米颗粒的理化性质表征是其毒性评估的前提

毒性研究中只需使用少量的纳米颗粒,这就要求所选用的纳米颗粒具有代表性,可以代表整体样品的性质。例如 Powers 等详细讨论了研究中粉末样品的取样、制样、常见错误以及解决办法[6]。在暴露前对纳米颗粒进行物理化学性质表征,在液体中分散或通过气溶胶形式分散的纳米颗粒,它们的性质会随着时间和周围环境的变化而变化,这些性质在进行毒性研究时也会不断发生改变。因此,在不同实验阶段对纳米颗粒的表征对于理解纳米颗粒的暴露特性非常重要。此外,纳米颗粒在干或湿的介质中都容易团聚,其尺寸、表面积、浓度和尺寸分布是毒理学评价的重要参数,需要根据实际暴露情况进行实时检测[7,8]。

2. 纳米颗粒在时间与空间变化时的性质表征

在纳米颗粒的生产或者供货环节对其进行表征是获得理化参数最直接和最易实现的方法,然而对于环境中的纳米颗粒,这些数据不能完全代表材料的特性,例如不能完全代表颗粒在空气中或在体内、体外生理环境中的特性。如果完全依赖初始的表征数据,将极大地限制结果的可比性和可信度。

对实验前、中、后三个阶段的纳米颗粒进行表征,可以为剂量-效应以及由材料特性所产生的作用提供高质量的数据支撑。其中实验后进行的表征尤为重要,因为它体现了实验前后纳米颗粒理化性质的变化,包括团聚、生物分子的物理吸附或化学吸附、表面化合物的变化等。因此,有必要增加实验后表征的数据。但在多数情况下,实验中进行的表征对于比较实验结果更为重要。

以下将详细介绍纳米颗粒的表征方法,目前面临的挑战是纳米颗粒成分通常含量较低,可能低于仪器的检测限;同时,还需要考虑纳米颗粒在空间及时间分辨率下的分布情况。

2.1.3　纳米颗粒理化性质

评估纳米颗粒风险前,需根据理化特性可能引起的结果确定要检测的理化参数种类,这需要多种表征方法联用来实现,以支持材料的质量控制、暴露、毒性和风险评估。通常在气溶胶暴露评估中使用的方法是检测纳米颗粒在工作场所和环境中的质量浓度,该方法使用抽气泵将样品抽滤到采样膜上进行测定,这不是评价纳米颗粒暴露的最好方法。纳米毒理学研究表明,质量浓度不是评估纳米颗粒吸入毒性的最适参数。目前环境领域设计的监测仪器适用于 PM_{10},$PM_{2.5}$ 和 $PM_{1.0}$ 等,不适用于精确检测空气动力学直径小于 $1~\mu m$ 的颗粒浓度。后续研发的监测仪器逐渐使用其他指标来表征纳米颗粒气溶胶,除质量浓度外,还包括纳米颗粒的数量和表面积,以及与颗粒形状相关的测量参数。

研究纳米颗粒毒性效应时,其理化性质对结果和结论具有关键作用。2005年,国际生命科学院研究基金会/风险科学院召集专家工作组,推荐了人造纳米材料风险评估中的理化性质参数种类,如颗粒的粒径、粒径分布、团聚状态、形状、晶体结构、化学组成、表面积、表面化学物质、表面电荷和多孔性[9]。随后,欧洲化学生态毒理学和毒理学会于2005年11月召开了旨在加强颗粒表征工作的研讨会,会议指出,众多理化参数可影响纳米颗粒的毒性,包括化学组成、溶解性、表面积和表面特性、粒径、粒径分布以及颗粒形状,这些参数在很大程度上决定了纳米材料的功能、毒理学和环境效应[10-12]。经济合作与发展组织（Organization for Economic Cooperation and Development，OECD)的人造纳米材料工作组于 2008 年提出了如下表征参数的建议：聚集/团聚，水溶性，含尘量，代表性的 TEM 照片，粒径分布，比表面积，Zeta 电位（表面电荷），表面化学（如适用），光催化活性，倾注密度（Pour Density），孔隙率，辛醇-水分配系数（相关的），氧化还原电位和自由基生成能力[13]。

　　纳米颗粒的理化特性参数有很多，需优先选择与毒理学、环境学最相关的理化特性参数，目前推荐选择的是粒径/粒径分布、聚集/团聚、纯度、表面积、表面化合物、结构、形状、溶解性、稳定性和表面电荷。各种表征方法都有其自身的局限性，必须依靠专业人员进行操作，通常需要联用多种表征方法对纳米颗粒进行表征，这就要求对不同表征结果或不同仪器产生的相同表征结果进行系统分析。

2.1.4　表征方法

　　随着科技进步，已经有一系列技术可用于纳米颗粒的表征，包括显微镜、光谱、分光光度计和色谱技术。表征技术的选择取决于纳米颗粒的种类以及对分辨率/表征质量的要求。这些技术还包括光声测量颗粒粒径，用断层扫描测定浓度和多相流动速度，光学捕获和原子力显微镜技术测量颗粒间的作用力，同轴成像技术结合图像分析测量颗粒形状。这些技术也提供了生产中在线检测的方法。显微镜在表征纳米结构特征和探测理化性质中发挥着重要作用，具体包括透射电子显微镜（Transmission Electron Microscope，TEM)、扫描电子显微镜（Scanning Electron Microscope，SEM)、扫描探针显微镜（Scanning Probe Microscope，SPM)、原子力显微镜（Atomic Force Microscope，AFM)和扫描近场光学显微镜（Scanning Near-Field Optical Microscope，SNOM)等。

1. 数量浓度

　　基于单颗粒光散射原理可直接检测空气中颗粒的数量浓度。常用的纳米气溶胶检测和计数仪器是凝聚核粒子计数器（Condensed Particle Counter，CPC)。CPC 使蒸汽冷凝在颗粒表面，使颗粒增大至能被光学检测的尺寸。CPC 检测的是颗粒数量浓度，但不能区分粒径大小，检测的粒径范围是 3～1000 nm。使用显微镜的图像处理技术可离线估算颗粒的数量浓度，包括 SEM 或 TEM。这样的图像处理同时可以提供粒径、形状、结构等信息。X 射线能谱仪（Energy Dispersive Spectrometer，EDS)还可提供颗粒的元素组成信息。

　　另一类仪器可以提供基于粒径分布的颗粒数量浓度信息，最常用的是扫描电迁移率粒径谱仪（Scanning Mobility Particle Sizer，SMPS)，它采用一种静电分级器来测量颗粒尺寸，并采用 CPC 来测定颗粒的浓度，粒径检测范围是 3～800 nm。

该仪器的不足是检测速度较慢,需要数分钟完成一次扫描,进而检测不同粒径范围的颗粒数量浓度。快速电迁移率粒径谱仪(Fast Mobility Particle Sizer,FMPS)可在一秒或更短的时间分辨率下进行检测,然而,当颗粒浓度较低时,SMPS 比 FMPS 灵敏度高。数量浓度的测定分析还可使用静电低压撞击器(Electrostatic Low Pressure Impactor,ELPI),测定范围是 $3\sim50$ nm,通过颗粒携带的电荷和有效表面积计算得到颗粒的数量浓度。该仪器可以同时收集颗粒,用于随后的离线分析。

2. 粒径

可使用多种方法检测和精确表征纳米颗粒的粒径、团聚状态及其在分散介质中的稳定性。有效测量颗粒物粒径分布的关键因素是良好的分散体系和足够多的颗粒数量,从而得到可信的数据统计结果。常用的方法包括动态光散射(Dynamic Light Scattering,DLS)、显微镜(如 SEM,TEM)和比表面积吸附等温线(Brunauer-Emmett-Teller,BET,也用来测量表面积)。其他一些特殊的、不常用的方法包括 X 射线、中子衍射技术、微分迁移率分析法和飞行时间质谱。场流分级法(Field Flow Fraction,FFF)是能够将纳米颗粒从混合物中分离出来的类似色谱的技术,它并不依靠纳米颗粒的化学组成,而是在一个正交力(根据仪器的配置有电、热、重力或者流动场)的作用下,根据主要层流所产生的流动性差异进行颗粒的分离。此分离方法不损坏样品,可用于后续的再分析。场流分离方法与在线检测器联用,如多角度激光散射(Multiangle Light Scattering,MALS)以及紫外光散射,可以测量纳米颗粒的粒径和浓度信息。对于一些特殊的纳米颗粒,例如金,使用紫外可见光谱(UV-Vis)能够得到粒径分布和团聚状态的准确信息。

对于存在于水介质中的纳米颗粒,动态光散射(DLS)是一种最常用的技术,可提供粒径和粒径分布信息,特别有利于毒性效应评估,因为它测定的是纳米颗粒在溶液中的尺寸,更符合液体暴露条件下的研究。然而,当颗粒分散状态不佳时,该技术则不再适用。通过 DLS 测得的粒径大小通常大于显微镜或 BET 测定结果,DLS 可以提供颗粒随时间和介质的改变,即悬浮稳定性特征。Dhawan 等在研究纳米颗粒的体外暴露毒性时,DLS 检测在其中起到重要作用[14,15]。此外,DLS 可以同时提供在不同溶液、不同 pH 和不同离子强度下的 Zeta 电位值。DLS 检测耗时少,成本低,可提供很好的统计学数据结果。DLS 技术的缺陷是不能区分由单个颗粒团聚形成的大颗粒和原本体积就很大的颗粒。对于干燥的粉末颗粒,SMPS 适用于检测能分散成气溶胶的材料,BET 等温吸附检测技术可以估算球形颗粒的平均粒径,BET 法同时还可直接测量样品的表面积、孔隙度,这些都是纳米颗粒表征中的重要参数。

显微镜是一种强大的分析技术,可提供尺寸、形状和形态信息。对于纳米颗粒,电子显微镜(最典型的是 SEM 和 TEM)能够提供高分辨率的图像,是唯一能在纳米尺度提供形状信息的技术。TEM 中的电子束在真空环境下穿透固体样品而产生放大图像和衍射图案,如果要求内部细节,则要求样本厚度小于 100～200 nm,较厚的样品可能需要更高的能量。TEM 分辨率通常是 0.5～3 nm,能够对晶格层和原子排列成像。若使用附加的探测器,如能谱,能得到空间分辨率小于 10 nm 的样品组分信息。

通常,电子显微镜分析的是干燥的固体样品,不是悬浮液样品。真空干燥会改变被测颗粒的大小和形状。用扫描电镜检测不导电的样品时,需要利用等离子体溅射仪在颗粒表面黏附一层导电材料,通常是金颗粒,厚度约几纳米,这个步骤可能会改变被测样品本身的性状。

图像质量对于样品分析至关重要。电子显微镜通常只提供二维图像,所以必须注意避免图像的偏移。受样品制备和分析条件的影响,高分辨显微镜可能产生假象结果,例如,TEM 检测要求高真空和薄膜样品,以使电子束穿透样品,当检测组织样品中的纳米颗粒时,需注意样品的保存、固定、染色等操作,从而保留样品细节信息并避免产生假象结果。

3. 形状

纳米颗粒可以呈现出不同的形状和结构,如球形、针形、管形、棒形、片层结构等。首先,形状可影响纳米颗粒在气相、液相中的迁移率和扩散速度,这是由于具有相同质量的球形和椭圆形颗粒之间的流体动力学半径不同(椭圆形更大)。其次,形状可影响颗粒沉积,并影响其在生物介质中的吸附动力学过程。

通常使用电子显微镜对纳米颗粒的形状、尺寸和团聚状态进行观察,如扫描探针显微镜(SPM),SPM 包括原子力显微镜和扫描隧道显微镜(Scanning Tunneling Microscope,STM),这些都是基于扫描探针(称为针尖)穿过有颗粒沉积的衬底,检测细小的差异,进而测定形状上的异同。SPM 技术可以在三个维度上检测单个纳米颗粒及其团聚颗粒,而 SEM 和 TEM 只有两个维度。与 SEM 和 TEM 类似,AFM 能够提供基于图像软件处理的粒径分布定量信息。另外,与 TEM 相比,AFM 适用于复杂环境下的测量工作,比如液体和固体环境。STM 图像能直接展示碳纳米管等复杂样品的三维形貌,同时还可以得到它们的原子结构和电子密度。

4. 团聚

纳米颗粒可在溶液、粉末和气相中发生团聚,这由颗粒尺寸、化学成分和表面电荷决定。此外,团聚还与生产、储存和处理条件有关,例如,即使通过气相反应新合成的碳纳米管,也会呈现出绳状或束状团聚的复合体形式。团聚状态可影响毒理学实验的结果,这直接由纳米分散体系的稳定性决定。振荡、超声波和/或表面活性剂常用于分散溶液中的纳米颗粒,可用于简单表征,若用于活体研究,这些过程或物质的加入可能会破坏细胞,并干扰毒性测试结果。如果干燥气溶胶颗粒发生团聚,就无法获得分散良好的气溶胶体系。通过与"理想"分散状态下的粒度分布进行对比,可对团聚程度进行定性评估。平均团聚数(Average Agglomeration Number,AAN)是指颗粒粒径中值体积与 BET 气体吸附平均等效球体积之比,用于评估团聚程度[16]。

5. 表面积

如前所述,在毒理学研究中,表面积是纳米颗粒的一个重要理化参数。纳米尺度的颗粒物表面积/体积比显著增加,大部分原子呈现在颗粒物表面而非内在的晶格内,与生物分子相互作用能力显著增加。气体吸附法被广泛用于比表面积的测定,氮气因其易获得性和良好的可逆吸附性,成为最常用的吸附质。BET 表面积表示可以与气体自由接触的表面积,根据比表面积和颗粒密度可计算得到初级颗粒直径(假定为等效球形直径)。虽然这种方法同时测量了粒径和表面积两个参数,但其缺点是以单分散的球形体系为假设,仅能提供平均粒径而不能提供粒径分布。

同位素表面积测定仪(Epiphaniometer)是另一种已成功用于直接测量气溶胶表面积的设备。在该设备中,气溶胶穿过充注室,衰减铜源上产生的铅同位素附着在颗粒物表面,随后通过毛细管被输送到收集滤波器,通过检测放射性物质剂量可以表示颗粒的总表面积。尽管同位素表面积测定仪已被成功地用于监测环境悬浮颗粒[17],但尚未广泛用于气溶胶暴露研究中,这可能是由于放射源使用方法较为复杂。此外,扩散荷电装置可直接测量气溶胶表面积。最近研发的纳米颗粒表面积检测仪可测量沉积在肺部的颗粒表面积(单位记作 mm^2/cm^3),测定原理是荷电的样品颗粒被收集在一个电绝缘的滤波器中,通过测量荷电速率得到沉积在肺部的颗粒表面积。这些新设备是已有纳米颗粒表征仪器的重要补充,在测量过程中,还需考虑气溶胶的原始电荷效应、材料组成、团聚状态及颗粒的形状等。另外,测量沉积颗粒表面积的优势尚需进一步研究。

6. 化学组成

化学组成,包括元素组成和化学结构,是所有材料的固有性质,也是影响纳米颗粒行为的重要参数。纳米颗粒具有多种化学组成,从无机组成,如金属(铁、镍、锌、钛、金、银、钯、铱和铂)和金属氧化物(氧化钛、氧化锌、二氧化硅、氧化铁等),到有机组成(富勒烯、碳纳米管、纳米聚合物、生物分子等)。化学纯度也是重要参数,因为一些纳米颗粒(例如碳纳米管)可能含有金属杂质,如铁、镍、钴,可能会干扰其毒性评估[12,18]。用于化学分析的电子能谱(Electron Spectroscopy for Chemical

Analysis,ESCA)、X 射线光电子能谱(X-ray Photoelectron Spectroscopy,XPS)和二次离子质谱法(Secondary Ion Mass Spectrometry,SIMS),已被广泛用于表征纳米颗粒的化学组成。此外,一些光谱技术包括电感耦合等离子体(ICP)技术、X 射线衍射(XRD)、核磁共振(NMR)、紫外-可见吸收光谱和荧光光谱都可用于检测特定的化学组分信息。

XPS 是一种非破坏性检测技术,适用于纳米材料表面元素的定量和定性分析,还可用于元素化学价态的研究,是目前应用最广泛的表面分析技术。XPS 必须采用超高真空系统,在通常情况下只能对固体样品进行分析,常用于金属纳米颗粒的表面分析,如铝、镍、金、碳纳米管以及核-壳结构的表面表征。差示扫描量热仪(Differential Scanning Calorimetry,DSC)在程序升温的条件下,测量试样与参比物之间的能量差随温度变化的一种分析方法,提供涉及吸热和放热过程的物理、化学变化的定性和定量信息。热重分析(Thermogravimetric Analysis,TGA)通过测定升温过程中样品的重量变化,提供纳米颗粒中存在的挥发性污染物或不稳定组分的信息。

电感耦合等离子体(ICP)和光学发射光谱(OES)联用或与质谱(MS)联用,具有很强的选择性及灵敏度,适于测定化学组分和所含微量杂质,样品在测定前需要完全溶解。这两种检测方法不能提供化学结构信息,对于轻质量元素的测定灵敏度较低。

气溶胶飞行时间质谱(Aerosol Time-of-flight Mass Spectrometry,ATOF-MS)是一种已商业化的检测技术,对纳米颗粒以气溶胶形式进行详细的化学组成分析,同时区分颗粒的大小,检测结果与 FFF 联用 TOF-MS 相似。

电子顺磁共振(Electron Paramagnetic Resonance,EPR)和电子自旋共振(Electron Spin Resonance,ESR)光谱用途广泛,属于非破坏性的定性和定量分析技术,可以提供材料的结构信息,如晶体缺陷和磁性特征,主要用于顺磁性元素和自由基的测定,在纳米科技领域已被用于金属纳米颗粒,如金、钯、镍、铁、锌氧化物和二氧化钛的表征。ESR 也可用于磁性纳米颗粒,如四氧化三铁的表征。

傅里叶变换红外光谱(Fourier Transform Infrared Spectroscopy,FTIR)和拉曼光谱(Raman Spectroscopy,RS)通过检测化学键的振动信息,对化学结构进行解析。FTIR 广泛用于富勒烯、碳纳米管、金属和金属氧化物纳米颗粒(如金、氧化锌)的结构分析。拉曼光谱是一种快速、非破坏性的方法,用来分析相变化(无定形或晶体)、尺寸变化和晶格应力。CNT 的结构信息和界面特性可以用 RS 来分析。

表面增强共振拉曼散射(Surface-Enhanced Resonant Raman Scattering,SERRS)是一种新兴的高通量单颗粒纳米分析技术,使用流动光谱,每秒能分析数百个纳米颗粒,通过测量瑞利和拉曼散射,根据其亮度和均匀性进行表征。已有研究表明,此项技术可以快速分析单个纳米颗粒,将在纳米科技领域被广泛应用[19]。

核磁共振（Nuclear Magnetic Resonance，NMR）是一种非破坏性技术。该技术可用于分析固体或液体样品，也可分析呈分散状的有机和无机纳米颗粒。NMR 也广泛用于研究纳米材料在动物体内的生物分布。例如，Faraj 等在大鼠模型中结合氟-3 和质子磁共振成像评估 SWCNT 纯化前、后的生物分布和生物效应[20]。

俄歇电子能谱（Auger Electron Spectroscopy，AES）可用于检测物质表面的元素组成，为纳米颗粒（如碳纳米管）和金属氧化物（如 TiO₂）提供化学组成的信息。

TEM 以及 SEM 结合能谱仪（Energy Dispersive Spectrometry，EDS）可以得到样品的元素组成信息。

7. 表面电荷

纳米颗粒分散在液体介质中，其表面荷电，电荷多少取决于颗粒的性质和周围介质。颗粒大小和表面电荷是影响纳米颗粒分散性的主要因素，还可影响其对离子、污染物和生物分子的吸附，以及细胞暴露效应。通常使用 Zeta 电位检测纳米颗粒的表面电荷，表征分散体系的稳定性。Zeta 电位通常在纯水中低浓度（1～10 mmol/L）低电解质含量下进行检测。滴定是用来寻找等电点的常用方法，其定义为 Zeta 电位是零时的 pH。通常情况下，除了 Zeta 电位（符号和幅度），材料的等电点在预期生理条件下（pH 和离子强度）也需要测定出来。纳米颗粒的 Zeta 电势通常通过光散射电泳或电声电泳方法测定。电势滴定也可用于获取颗粒表面电荷信息。颗粒表面官能团的 pK_a 值可用颗粒表面电荷密度来确定。

8. 晶体结构

具有相同化学组分的材料可能具有不同的晶体结构，并且表现出迥异的物理化学性质。一些无机纳米颗粒的结构研究显示，由于表面原子相对晶格具有非常大的比例，晶格类型可对纳米颗粒的整体结构有重要影响。尺寸减小可能产生不连续的晶面即增加结构缺陷的数量，以及扰乱材料的电子结构，随之会导致毒性的产生。XRD 常被用于研究纳米颗粒的表面原子结构（如晶体结构、晶格缺陷）。TEM 还可提供晶体结构信息，如表面原子排列和原子尺度上的缺陷。结合能谱仪（EDS）可以得到样品的元素信息。

2.1.5　总结

毒性评估前纳米颗粒理化性质系统表征方法的研究已经取得了一定的进展，多种表征方法联用可更加科学地描述纳米颗粒的真实状态，是评估纳米颗粒生物效应的重要组成部分[21]。合适和通用的表征方法是结果可重复性的重要保障，同时还为阐释纳米颗粒的生物效应提供了大量基础数据。但需要指出的是，一些影响纳米颗粒生物活性的关键参数，仍是未知或者尚待深入探讨。因此，材料表征应遵从全面和广泛的原则。如果发现某种材料毒性大但研究前后并没有进行理化性质表征,这样的研究不具有科学价值。

材料的完整表征是耗时、昂贵和复杂的,并且难以被完全表征。在一定程度上,表征参数与研究目标有关。目前,在毒性研究中普遍认同基本表征参数,如粒径、形状、化学组成、分散状态、表面积和表面化学等是必需的。

2.2　纳米颗粒的聚集与团聚

纳米颗粒通常是以聚集或团聚的形式存在于环境中,颗粒间的紧密结合程度决定了是属于聚集(Aggregation)还是团聚(Agglomeration),聚集是颗粒间紧密结合,团聚是范德华力的弱相互作用。团聚和聚集在一起的颗粒可以是相同的也可以是不同的颗粒,因此,颗粒表面可能会受到不同的作用而发生改变。

当颗粒尺寸小至纳米尺度时,其理化性质将会发生变化,甚至呈现出新的特性,比如,当二氧化钛尺寸小于 50 nm 时,颜色将不再是白色而变成无色,一些绝缘材料,在纳米尺度时可以导电,一些难溶的颗粒在小于 100 nm 时溶解性增加。

纳米颗粒类似于气体或蒸汽,在空气中的运动行为与颗粒大小、颗粒的形成机制及扩散力有关,对于小于 100 nm 的颗粒,扩散是颗粒运动的主要方式,扩散速度取决于扩散系数,与颗粒大小负相关。纳米颗粒比微米颗粒扩散得更快,因此,纳米颗粒在工厂环境中可以从生产位置快速迁移至很远距离,影响远处的空气环境。在扩散与布朗运动的共同作用下,纳米颗粒在空气中发生碰撞,导致聚集和团聚,形成大尺寸颗粒物,尺寸大小取决于纳米颗粒的数量浓度和迁移率,迁移率与直径成反比。

低浓度的纳米颗粒也会发生团聚,粒径为 1～100 nm 的颗粒团聚的很快,粒径从 100 nm 左右增长至 2 μm 时,团聚将较缓慢,从 100 nm 至 2 μm 称为"蓄积模式"(Accumulation Mode)。最初气溶胶颗粒相互接近,并接触,形成较为松散的大颗粒或团聚物,气溶胶团聚过程是从颗粒之间的布朗运动或热力学运动开始,这在气溶胶中是很常见的现象。如果相对运动是由外力作用所致,如重力、介电或空气动力学等,这个过程就被称为"动力学团聚"。

重力学沉降是指颗粒由于重力作用沉降到其他介质中,沉降速度取决于颗粒直径及沉降过程中气流的性质,尤其是摩擦系数。对于大颗粒,摩擦系数可以忽略,而颗粒越小,摩擦系数的影响将越大,这体现在热力学位移与重力位移之间的比值,对于 10 nm 的颗粒,比值是 4800(主要是扩散,可以忽略沉降)。总之,对于小颗粒尤其纳米颗粒,重力沉降并不是重要影响因素。

纳米颗粒从粉末形成气溶胶是个复杂的过程,影响这一过程的因素有很多,包括大小、形状、静电荷及环境湿度。作用力导致颗粒间相互团聚,同样也会导致颗粒吸附到其他物质的表面上,颗粒越小,就越难从吸附的表面上脱离形成分散的气溶胶颗粒。对于大多数纳米材料,一旦发生聚集或团聚,就很难分开或形成分散状态。

颗粒表面和界面性质对纳米尺度材料十分重要,随着尺寸减小,颗粒表面的原子数比颗粒内部的原子数显著增加,颗粒活性增大,颗粒表面的活性基团能够改变其毒理学性质。

纳米材料的生物效应取决于纳米颗粒的物理化学性质,与相同化学组成的宏观尺寸材料相比,纳米材料可能会产生不同的健康影响。因此,在风险评估中,纳米颗粒的物理化学性质包括颗粒尺寸分布、表面化学及水溶液中的颗粒活性都尤其重要。表 2.1 列出与纳米颗粒相关的理化性质。

表 2.1   与纳米颗粒相关的理化性质

性质	注释
形状	物理形状及颗粒形态,包含纳米表面结构形状
表面积	颗粒与生物界面相接触的表面积(生物相关颗粒表面积)
表面化学	与颗粒生物活性相关的表面化学
组成	颗粒化学组成
核心与表面组成的均一性	颗粒核与表面组成之间系统性差异
组成分布的不均一性	纳米颗粒间组成的不均一性
溶解性	纳米材料在特定的生物环境下的溶解速度,或纳米材料特定组成成分在溶解过程中的释放
电荷(生物体液中)	在肺气管内沉积后颗粒的电荷
晶型	纳米颗粒的晶体结构
多孔性	纳米颗粒内部的多孔程度
沉积后颗粒大小和/或结构的改变情况	颗粒解聚或塌陷后颗粒大小及/或结构的变化,包括纳米结构的塌陷或者致密结构的扩展变化
沉积后颗粒组分的释放情况	在肺气管沉积后从颗粒或其团聚体中快速释放出来的化学成分
刺激性	依赖于外在刺激效应的生物活性,如光或磁场作用
对环境的功能响应	依赖于内在生物环境的生物活性,可随内在环境变化

从表 2.1 可知,纳米颗粒毒性评估中没有简单通用的理化参数,需要进行全面的理化性质表征,但这需要投入很大的工作量。如下列出了毒理学研究中必须表征的理化参数:

◇ 颗粒尺寸

◇ 尺寸分布

◇ 表面积

◇ 晶型

◇ 表面活性

◇ 表面组成

◇ 纯度

在进行风险评估时需对如下理化参数进行表征：

◇ 晶体结构/结晶度

◇ 在相关介质中的团聚程度

◇ 组分/表面包被

◇ 表面活性

◇ 纳米材料合成和/或制备方法，包括合成后的修饰

◇ 样品纯度

◇ 根据暴露途径，利用相关媒介表征颗粒大小及大小分布（液体介质状态），表面积（干燥状态）性质。

　　除了上述应该表征的参数，如下参数也尽可能检测：形状、Zeta 电位及疏水性。另外，在进行呼吸相关的风险评估时，可以通过测定含尘量（Dustiness）确定纳米颗粒在空气中的最大分散量，这种检测方法如果能够标准化，将可以提供各种粉尘颗粒的含尘指数，进而评估粉尘操作时的危险性。部分常规分析技术可以根据纳米颗粒的特点进行修正以用于纳米颗粒的表征分析，但多数理化性质参数还是需要特定的技术方法进行分析。

第 3 章　纳米颗粒暴露途径与暴露事件

3.1　引　　言

3.1.1　暴露

化学试剂暴露可能会对个体或人群产生潜在健康风险,通常认为随着剂量的增加,有害物质在生物体内蓄积量增大,对机体造成损伤。为了进行风险控制,通常主要关注暴露剂量。国际暴露分析协会(The International Society of Exposure Science,ISES)将暴露定义为"剂量与靶标之间的关系",即在一个暴露周期内将人类作为暴露靶标研究其受暴露程度。辨识和控制暴露在风险评估和防护中至关重要。暴露评估需要确定暴露剂量、时间以及经受暴露的人群数量。因此,暴露通常是研究(定量或估算)在一个阶段内的暴露强度(浓度)和持续时间(或频率)。控制暴露(为零)可有效地消除有毒物质的暴露风险,没有暴露就没有风险。产业工人的主要暴露途径是经呼吸道吸入,经口摄入以及皮肤接触渗透。

大气悬浮颗粒物进入工人体内的主要途径是经呼吸道吸入,一旦进入人体,颗粒将可能沉积在整个呼吸道,沉积位置和沉积数量取决于颗粒尺寸。经口摄入途径可能是因为手与口的接触,或通过吸吮或舔舐受过污染的器皿,或经口摄入受污染的食物,也可能是吞咽从肺部代谢出来的含有颗粒物的黏液。目前关于职业暴露的研究很少。

工作场所中皮肤暴露途径逐渐受到关注。工人的皮肤可能会在操作过程中接触纳米材料或皮肤表面被纳米材料污染而发生暴露。控制皮肤暴露的措施是佩戴皮肤防护装备,如手套,这需要保证防护装备本身不是污染源,不存在暴露风险。

3.1.2　纳米颗粒的潜在暴露

人造纳米材料可通过职业暴露、环境效应和消费者接触对人类造成潜在暴露。产业工人的暴露可能发生在纳米材料的整个生命周期。在纳米材料的研发阶段,因产量较小,且实验条件控制严格,即使发生泄漏等突发事故,也只有很少部分的人暴露于纳米材料。纳米材料的商业化生产阶段,材料的合成、包装、运输、贮存等生产环节均可发生暴露,且暴露剂量较大。现代工业中使用纳米材料的行业详见表 3.1,生产或使用纳米产品均可引起潜在暴露,这些产品也包括纳米复合材料。纳米材料最后可能通过焚烧、粉碎或研磨等方式结束其生命周期,进入环境,通过大气、土壤、水体等生态循环系统对人类产生潜在影响。因此,对于某种纳米颗粒,其会不会发生暴露,主要取决于制造、使用和处理这些材料的具体过程;同时,发生暴露的水平、持续时间,甚至所生产加工材料的性质,都与发生暴露后可能形成的危害程度直接相关。

表 3.1　典型纳米颗粒的应用

应用领域	材料		
	富勒烯(C_{60},C_{70},C_{80},衍生物)	碳纳米管(SWCNT和MWCNT)	金属及其氧化物
存储氢能	√	√	
环境修复			√
催化作用			√
药物输送	√	√	√
医学成像	√	√	
疾病治疗	√	√	
光伏电池	√	√	√
纺织业		√	
增强复合材料		√	
电子工业和电子器件			
光学器件	√		√
涂料和颜料	√	√	√
化妆品			√
陶瓷工业		√	
抗氧化剂	√		√
润滑油	√		√
传感器和相关器件			
吸附剂		√	√
能量学		√	√
磁力学			√
水的纯化和过滤			
气体减排			√
天然绿色产品			
量子计算		√	√
建筑业			√
光电子学器件		√	
表面活性剂	√		

3.1.3 暴露评估指标

早期煤炭行业流行病学研究中,使用光学显微镜对沉积在过滤膜上的颗粒进行计数作为评价分析方法[22],这是一种粗略的使用颗粒计数法评估暴露水平的方法,表示为每 cc(cm^3)或每 m^3 空气中有多少个颗粒。后期的流行病学研究发现,尘肺病与质量浓度有很好的相关性,表示为 mg/m^3,具体方法是使用含有过滤膜的采样仪器收集颗粒物,通过对过滤膜采样前、后进行称重,计算质量差值,以质量浓度表示作为暴露评价方法。因为质量浓度评估更为客观,所以成为多种危险化学品和颗粒物暴露程度的标准表示方法。特例情况是对纤维样品的暴露限值表示为纤维数量浓度,例如石棉纤维。

在纳米安全性监测及评价领域,现有三个暴露评估指标,分别是:①质量浓度(单位:mg/m^3);②数量浓度(单位:m^3);③表面积浓度(单位:m^2/m^3)。与质量浓度相比,毒理学研究认为纳米颗粒的毒性与表面积浓度更为相关。而根据大气颗粒物污染加重了人类呼吸道疾病的恶化、心血管病人死亡人数的增加和老年人呼吸道疾病病例的增加等研究结果,研究人员认为颗粒数量可作为纳米颗粒暴露评估指标[23]。上述三个指标代表不同的意义,所以建议在纳米安全性评价工作中,需要同时测量这三个暴露指标[24]。

3.2 工作场所暴露途径

工作场所中纳米颗粒可能通过呼吸道吸入、皮肤接触以及食道摄入进入体内。人体暴露水平通常可以定义为对某种物质的摄入量,在皮肤暴露时取决于皮肤的接触总量,而在呼吸暴露时则指吸入物质的总量,通常与工人呼吸区该物质在空气中的浓度成正比。暴露可能是单次暴露,也可能是一系列重复暴露或者连续暴露。在暴露评估中,不论是通过实验测定还是计算机模拟,除了要考虑暴露水平,还需要考虑暴露时间、暴露频率以及引起的急性和慢性反应、局部和系统效应。

3.2.1 呼吸暴露

对于许多物质和暴露场所,呼吸道吸入是主要的暴露途径。呼吸暴露的主要参数是在一定时间内,呼吸区的平均颗粒浓度数。当用于比较一个连续的或周期性的暴露事件时,通常采用 8 小时作为一个周期。当有些物质存在短期暴露引起急性健康效应的可能时,则也可以评价短期内产生暴露的情况。以特定工作为对象的暴露评估,可以在不同的时间段进行。呼吸暴露可能来源于气体、蒸汽或者大气环境中的气溶胶,液体及固体成分(包括废气、尘埃、纤维)。精准的气溶胶暴露表征是很困难的,这是因为气溶胶中的颗粒大小随着时间和空间会发生改变,并影响通过呼吸道或消化道进入人体的程度。呼吸暴露可以通过质量浓度、暴露时间和频率来定义,通常表示为 ppm(百万分之一)或吸入的每单位空气体积,平均暴露剂量浓度,例如,mg/m³ 8 小时,时间加权平均值(Time-Weighted Average,TWA)。

3.2.2　皮肤暴露

皮肤可能是某些特定物质或者暴露条件的主要暴露途径,这些物质主要对皮肤有局部作用,或具有穿透皮肤进入机体的能力。通常采用如下两个术语描述皮肤暴露。

◇ 潜在皮肤暴露:用于评估黏附在工作服外面及皮肤表面的污染物的量,是身体各部分暴露评估的总和,包括手和足。潜在皮肤暴露是最常用的评估指标。

◇ 实际皮肤暴露:用于评估实际接触皮肤的污染物的量。该数据受到防护服防护效果的影响,规范的管理制度可以明显减少实际皮肤暴露量。

局部高浓度的污染物可能会引起皮肤暴露,例如,搅拌、装载、喷涂或者高浓度的气溶胶环境,都有可能使手部皮肤或衣服上黏附污染物,影响暴露量的因素包括污染物的数量和浓度、皮肤面积和部位(如面部皮肤比手部皮肤的吸收量高)、皮肤质地特点、暴露时间和频率、人群特点、是否存在促吸收物质等。皮肤接触污染物的主要途径包括空气沉积,直接接触(如浸入、泼溅)以及与黏附污染物的物体表面接触。污染物从手部转移到身体其他部位是皮肤暴露的重要组成部分。当用手脱去工作服或其他个人防护装备时,也会引起暴露。皮肤暴露量以单位面积污染物含量表示。

3.2.3　经口摄入

工作场所中口与黏附污染物的手之间无意识接触可能引起经口摄入污染物,或使用被污染的餐具、食用被污染的食物等都可能引起经口摄入污染物,这些暴露可以通过规范的管理制度、完善的防护措施和良好的卫生习惯减少发生的可能性,如将工作区与休息区分离,设立更衣区、清洗区等。

3.3　典型纳米材料生产场所暴露评估

3.3.1　现场纳米颗粒暴露种类

与纳米材料的种类相比,关于生产场所纳米颗粒暴露评估的数据还较少,表3.2 对已有研究进行了汇总。这些研究主要针对检测相关的暴露数据,其中两项研究分别报道了呼吸暴露途径和皮肤暴露途径,目前还没有经口摄入途径的研究。上述大部分的研究结果出自大学或研究所,较少一部分由企业发表,通常使用多种方法主要检测了纳米颗粒的数量浓度、质量浓度和尺寸分布,只有一项研究直接测量纳米颗粒的表面积浓度。本指南选取产量大、应用广泛的碳纳米管和二氧化钛纳米颗粒进行重点阐述。

表 3.2　现有纳米颗粒暴露评估研究报告

第一作者(文献)	碳纳米管	富勒烯	金属	金属氧化物
Maynard[25]	单壁碳纳米管			
Methner[26]	碳纳米纤维			
Han[27]	多壁碳纳米管			
Bello[28]	多壁碳纳米管			
Bello[20]	多壁碳纳米管			
Fujitani[29]		混合物		
Yeganeh[30]	混合物	混合物		
Hsu[31]				二氧化钛
Demou[32]			金属	金属氧化物
Peters[33]				LiTiO$_x$
Tsai[34]			银	氧化铝

3.3.2　碳纳米管暴露及其风险评估

碳纳米管(CNT)作为一种纳米材料,主要由呈六边形排列的碳原子构成数层到数十层的同轴圆管。单层结构的碳纳米管称为单壁碳纳米管(SWCNT),多层结构的称为多壁碳纳米管(MWCNT),层与层之间保持固定的距离,约 0.34 nm,直径一般为 2~20 nm。具有许多新颖的力学、电学和化学性能。近些年随着碳纳米管及纳米材料研究的深入,其广阔的应用前景也不断地展现出来,据估计,在接下来的十年,碳纳米管的产量将有一个稳定的增长[35]。大规模生产意味着职业暴露风险的增加。

1. 暴露风险

已有研究表明,CNT 在转移、称量、调配、散装粉的混合以及对 CNT 复合材料的切割和钻孔等操作时会发生释放。Maynard 等首次评估了 SWCNT 生产现场的颗粒释放,当缺乏控制措施时,SWCNT 释放量是 0.7~53 μg/m^3,尺寸大于 1 μm,操作工人手套上的 SWCNT 黏附量是 217~6020 μg[25]。Han 等发现释放的颗粒物中只有一小部分是 MWCNT,没有控制措施时,释放的总颗粒物浓度是 0.21~

$0.43\ mg/m^3$，释放的 MWCNT 数量浓度是 $172.9\sim193.6$ 个$/cm^3$，实施控制措施后，MWCNT 数量浓度下降至 $0.018\sim0.05$ 个$/cm^3$，检测不到总颗粒物的质量浓度[27]。Bello 等使用快速迁移率粒径谱仪（Fast Mobility Particle Sizer，FMPS）和凝结核粒子计数器（CPC）实时在线检测了生产过程中释放的 MWCNT 数量浓度[28]，结果表明生产过程中空气颗粒总浓度没有增加，电子显微镜下也没有观察到 MWCNT。然而，这项研究并没有提供能够区别背景颗粒物和 MWCNT 的数据。CPC 3007（测量范围 10 nm～1 μm）检测没有通风控制的室内环境的总颗粒数量浓度范围是 $2000\sim10000$ 个$/cm^3$，该项研究中 CPC 3007 测量值是 $4000\sim7000$ 个$/cm^3$，有可能源自环境中如森林火灾、交通、燃烧等产生的悬浮颗粒物。

　　CNT 生产过程中释放的颗粒主要是碳材料和金属催化剂颗粒，其形态和化学成分不同于人造纳米颗粒。为了评估人造纳米颗粒暴露风险，需要区分不同加工工艺流程释放的纳米颗粒。我们检测了 CNT 生产处理流程中纳米颗粒的释放，包括 CNT 薄膜在硅衬底上生长后的激光标记步骤，从硅衬底旋转分离的过程，这些检测工作都在洁净的 CNT 生产车间中开展，洁净间采用向下排风的方式，检测结果见图 3.1，两个 CNT 处理过程都瞬间释放少量颗粒物，但在呼吸区域检测不到纳米颗粒的释放，这说明通风设备能够快速清除释放的纳米颗粒。

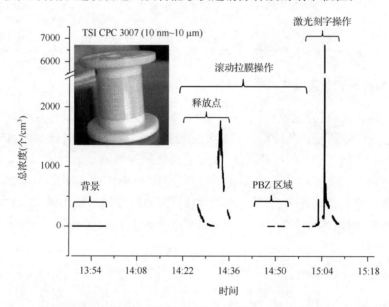

图 3.1　使用 CPC 3007 颗粒计数器检测 CNT 加工车间中释放的颗粒物数量浓度，内嵌图显示拉丝生产的 CNT 产品，距离释放源 10 cm

　　化学气相沉积法（CVD）可制备多种类型的 CNT，Tsai 等研究了实验室通风橱中气体颗粒物和 CNT 的释放水平[36]。环境背景中颗粒物浓度的测定有助于评估 CNT 的释放水平。在通风橱中检测了 SWCNT 的释放数量浓度,峰值为 $4 \times 10^6 \sim 1 \times 10^7$ 个/cm³,平均粒径为 50 nm。工人呼吸区域的颗粒物浓度很低 (<2000 个/cm³)。Methner 等在生产或使用碳纳米管和碳纳米纤维(CNF)的不同场所进行了释放和暴露评估研究,结果表明短期使用 SWCNT 或 CNF,不会造成暴露[37,38]。呼吸区域的最高浓度(38 μg/m³)出现在从反应器中收集 SWCNT 的工序过程,尽管元素碳(EC)的浓度低于检测限,但大部分收集的样本通过电子显微镜观察证明了 SWCNT 或 CNF 暴露的发生。Dahm 等比较了 MWCNT, SWCNT,CNF 材料初级生产过程和二级加工过程之间的暴露水平[39],处理干粉的两个二级生产设备的呼吸区域的颗粒物浓度比所有的初级生产区域都高,显微镜观察所有区域收集的样品,均发现 CNT/CNF,其中二级加工区域的 CNT/CNF 数量最高。随后,Dahm 等继续对 CNT、CNF 的制造商和使用者进行了暴露评估[40],可吸入 EC 在呼吸区域的浓度范围是 $0.02 \sim 2.94$ μg/m³,其几何平均数 (GM)为 0.34 μg/m³,8 小时时间加权平均浓度为 0.16 μg/m³。EC 在呼吸区域的可吸入体积分数范围是 $0.01 \sim 79.57$ μg/m³,其 GM 为 1.21 μg/m³。TEM 中最常见的 CNT 是直径 $2 \sim 5$ μm 的团聚体以及 >5 μm 的团聚体。该调查表明,EC 在呼吸区域的时间加权平均浓度低于 NIOSH 建议的阈值(96%<1 μg/m³,可吸入体积分数),同时 30% 的可吸入体积分数>1 μg/m³。研究人员建议联合使用 EC 监测(包括呼吸道和可吸入体积分数)和 TEM 观察以更好地评估纳米颗粒暴露水平。

目前,已有少量关于含碳纳米管复合材料的切割、钻孔和磨光过程中纳米颗粒释放水平的研究[20,41,42],科研人员采用 NIOSH 发布的"7400 方法"测定纤维浓度,结果表明切割过程中颗粒的释放随着复合样品厚度(或层数)的增加而增加,钻孔、高速打孔和更大的钻孔机产生的颗粒物数量浓度更高,在加工过程中使用润滑剂可以大大减少切割和打孔时颗粒物的释放量;随着复合材料厚度的增加,需要更高的输入能量(如更高的钻头转速,较大的钻头)和更长的钻孔时间,从而引起颗粒物释放水平的增高,并且钻孔比切割更容易产生纳米颗粒;磨光操作产生的颗粒物数量最少,可以忽略不计。TEM 观察表明磨光操作产生的突出形态的 CNT 是微米尺度,与团聚产生的相同尺度的 CNT 显著不同。

综上所述,研究人员采用多种检测方法和指标证明了 CNT 生产场所中纳米颗粒的释放(表 3.3)。与质量浓度和数量浓度相比,元素碳检测是一个更实用、灵敏的暴露指标。目前关于碳纳米管的暴露数据较少,大多数研究是在没有或缺少防护措施的情况下进行的,在线监测和离线分析联用,可以提供纳米颗粒高浓度释放时的定量数据和形态学图像。

表3.3　呼吸区域颗粒物释放浓度汇总

暴露评估指标	呼吸区域颗粒物释放浓度	参考文献
可吸入组分质量浓度($\mu g/m^3$)	0.7~53	Maynard et al. 2004[25]
总质量浓度($\mu g/m^3$)	N.D.~430	Han et al. 2008[27]
总质量浓度($\mu g/m^3$)	7.8~320.8	Lee et al. 2010[113]
可吸入组分元素碳($\mu g/m^3$)	64~1094	Methner et al. 2010[38]
可吸入组分元素碳($\mu g/m^3$)	N.D.~38	Methner et al. 2012[50]
可吸入组分元素碳($\mu g/m^3$)	N.D.~7.86	Dahm et al. 2012[39]
可吸入组分元素碳($\mu g/m^3$)	45~80	Birch et al. 2011[114]
总颗粒物数量浓度(个/cm^3,P/B)	4000~7000,≈1	Bello et al. 2008[28]
总颗粒物数量浓度(个/cm^3,P/B)	<2000,≈1	Tsai et al. 2009[115]
总质量浓度(PM_{10},$\mu g/m^3$)	800~2400	Bello et al. 2009[20]
纤维浓度(fibers/cm^3)	0.2	Bello et al. 2009[20]
纤维浓度(fibers/cm^3)	1.9	Bello et al. 2010[41]
打磨工艺释放总颗粒物质量浓度($\mu g/m^3$,P/B)	0.2~21.4, 0.66~24.4	Cena and Peters. 2011[56]
打磨工艺释放总颗粒物数量浓度与背景浓度比值	1.04	Cena and Peters. 2011[56]
称量过程,总质量浓度($\mu g/m^3$,P/B)	N.D.~0.03,1.79	Cena and Peters. 2011[56]
打磨工艺释放总颗粒物数量浓度与背景浓度比值	1.06	Cena and Peters. 2011[56]
可吸入组分元素碳($\mu g/m^3$)	0.02~2.94	Dahm et al. 2015[40]
纤维浓度(fibers/cm^3)	0.017~0.06	Fonseca et al. 2015[116]
可吸入组分元素碳($\mu g/m^3$)	6.2~9.3	Lee et al. 2015[117]
可吸入粉尘质量浓度($\mu g/m^3$)	73~93	Hedmer et al. 2014[118]
可吸入组分元素碳($\mu g/m^3$)	0.08~7.4	Hedmer et al. 2014[118]
可吸入组分元素碳纤维浓度(fibers/cm^3)	0.04~2.0	Hedmer et al. 2014[118]

注：N.D. 表示未检测到颗粒物；

P/B 表示与背景的比值

2. 暴露评估参数

工作场所纳米颗粒暴露评估常用的三个主要参数是质量浓度(单位:mg/m³),数量浓度(单位:个/m³)及表面积浓度(单位:m²/m³)。对于相同质量浓度的颗粒物,当粒径减小到 100 nm 以下时,数量浓度和表面积浓度随粒径减小呈指数级增加,所以数量浓度和表面积浓度是现场暴露评估中两个更重要的指标。此外,已有研究表明,纳米颗粒暴露引起健康效应可能与表面积浓度具有更好的相关性,而非质量浓度。此外,元素碳(Elemental Carbon,EC)的质量浓度被推荐作为碳纳米管的职业暴露控制阈值(Occupational Exposure Limit,OEL)。然而,EC 的质量浓度和可吸入粉尘总量的浓度仍然不能直接表示碳纳米管的暴露量,所以研究中通常使用暴露值与背景值的比值(P/B)评价纳米颗粒的暴露水平。碳纳米管产生的毒性还与合成材料时使用的金属催化剂有关,所以还应采用 ICP-MS 等技术对CNT 的化学组分进行测定。

3. 职业暴露阈值

截至目前,国际上尚未发布公认的碳纳米颗粒职业暴露阈值。德国职业安全与健康研究所(IFA)推荐使用颗粒数量浓度作为监测碳纳米颗粒释放的基准参数(表 3.4),按照尺寸、化学组分、生物持久性、密度将纳米材料分成四组,对低密度(<6000 kg/m³)和高密度(>6000 kg/m³)纳米颗粒,假设纳米材料是球形的(直径<100 nm),建议质量浓度阈值为 0.1 mg/m³。NIOSH 于 2011 年 4 月推荐的TiO₂ 接触限值是 0.3 mg/m³(超细与纳米级 TiO₂-NIDSH)和 2.4 mg/m³(细TiO₂-NIOSH)。碳纳米管可能表现出类似石棉的效应,因此可使用石棉的职业暴露阈值。

表 3.4　四类纳米颗粒职业暴露阈值(8 小时时间加权平均浓度)

分类	描述	密度	推荐职业接触限值(8 小时时间加权平均浓度)	举例
1	质地坚硬难降解的纤维状物质,产生类似于石棉纤维的效应	—	0.01 fibers/cm³	碳纳米管
	元素碳(NIOSH)	—	1 μg/m³	碳纳米管
2	介于 1~100 nm 之间难降解的颗粒状纳米材料	>6000 kg/m³	20000 particles/cm³ 0.1 mg/m³	Ag, Au, CeO₂, CoO, Fe, Fe$_x$O$_y$, La, Pb, Sb₂O₅, SnO₂

续表

分类	描述	密度	推荐职业接触限值 （8 小时时间加 权平均浓度）	举例
3	介于 1～100 nm 之间难降解的颗粒状纳米材料	＜6000 kg/m³	40000 particles/cm³ 0.1 mg/m³ 0.3 mg/m³（超细与 纳米级 TiO₂-NIOSH）	Al_2O_3，SiO_2， TiN，TiO_2，ZnO， 纳米黏土，炭黑，C_{60}，树 枝状大分子，聚苯乙烯
4	介于 1～100 nm 之间生物可降解的颗粒状纳米材料	—	适用的职业 暴露限值	脂肪颗粒，盐类颗粒物质

注：摘自 2012 年召开的荷兰社会经济会议

4. 暴露评估策略

危险源辨识和防护措施在风险评估和管理中至关重要，暴露评估可用于识别释放的纳米颗粒和论证防护措施的有效性，所以需要选择合理的评估方案以保护人类健康和环境安全。我们依据已有研究结果，建立了适用于纳米颗粒的暴露评估策略（图 3.2），由分层递进的方法执行职业暴露评估，如果检测到纳米颗粒则继续更高层级的评估。第一步是收集基本信息并确认生产场所是存在纳米颗粒释放

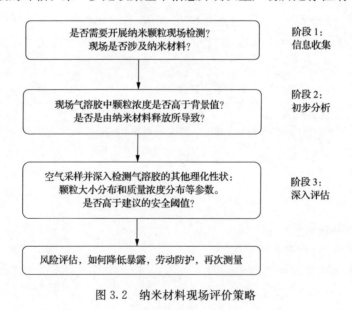

图 3.2　纳米材料现场评价策略

条件,并论证这种潜在风险是否可以被排除。第二步是测量颗粒数量浓度并进行相关释放源的电镜分析检测。碳纳米材料的质量浓度可以根据 NIOSH 的方法5040 进行测定。配有 EDS 的 TEM 可以验证碳纳米材料的存在。同时应详细记录通风设施、防护设备、工人数量、暴露频率等相关信息。如果确认存在纳米颗粒的释放,则在第三步中进行更深入、详细的暴露检测,包括粒径分布,质量浓度、呼吸区域中的元素碳质量浓度、纤维数量浓度、表面积浓度以及电子显微镜分析。

3.3.3　富勒烯暴露及其风险评估

富勒烯(Fullerene)是单质碳的第三种同素异形体,另两种同素异形体分别是石墨与金刚石。富勒烯指的是一类物质,任何由碳一种元素组成,以球状、椭圆状或管状结构存在的物质,都可以被称作富勒烯。其中,形状似足球一样的 C_{60} 最为人所熟知。很多研究表明,富勒烯类化合物在抗艾滋病病毒、抗肿瘤、酶活性抑制、光动力学治疗等方面有着独特的生物学功能。

到目前为止,只有两个研究组报道了富勒烯的相关暴露数据。这些数据见表 3.5。

表 3.5　与富勒烯相关的研究结果总结

环境		活动						参考文献
生产场所	实验室	合成	包装	清洗	加工	搅拌	切割	
♯			E	E		E		[29]
♯		0	E	E				[30]

注:♯表示环境监测;
　　E 表示存在明显的释放暴露;
　　0 表示监测但无明显释放暴露

Fujitani 等测量了日本生产富勒烯的工厂的空气中富勒烯的理化性质、悬浮颗粒的数量浓度和数量大小分布[29]。在生产设备中,利用溶剂萃取的方法,将混合富勒烯从碳氢化合物和氧气混合燃烧产生的烟尘中萃取出来。混合富勒烯的产物中包括 C_{60},C_{70} 和其他更多碳原子组成的富勒烯。富勒烯产品主要是以粒子聚集体或团聚的形成存在,混合富勒烯颗粒的直径大约为 20 μm。这家工厂的生产能力为 40 吨/年。富勒烯生产在一个密闭的系统里,旨在减少生产过程中潜在的暴露风险。干燥以后,富勒烯被转运到一个储罐中进行储存,直到被移走和袋装。在包装过程中会使用一个真空吸尘器用于除去粉尘。一定量的富勒烯装袋后,在同一个房间里进行称重。

数量和体积分布结果,包括不同时间的分布结果,使一系列的生产活动能够相互比较,如不开工,装袋,使用真空吸尘器和温和的搅拌。根据时间序列,结果可分为四个尺寸范围:10~50 nm,50~100 nm,100~2000 nm 和>2000 nm。材料源头、工人和测量仪器的相互距离都在 1.5 m 的范围内。在这个设备里面只进行了一天的测试,第二天在设备的外面对环境条件进行了测量。表 3.6 显示的是从论文中提取出来的数据(精确度有限)。注意测量浓度的变化并没有立即发生在活动的开始,所以这里报道的数字是在活动发生后上升至最高水平时的浓度。

表 3.6　从 Fujitani 等[29] 报道文章中提取出来的数据

尺寸范围 (nm)	颗粒数量浓度(颗粒/cm³)				估算的体积浓度($\times 10^9$ nm³/cm³)			
	10~50	50~100	100~2000	>2000	10~50	50~100	100~2000	>2000
不开工时室内的空气浓度	10000	7000	3000	0	0.1	2	10	10
开始回收和装袋	15000	7000	3000	0	0.2	2	10	50
结束包装,工人离开后	10000	7000	3000	0	0.1	2	10	10
开始抽真空	15000	7000	3000	0	0.3	2	10	30
开始温和搅拌	10000	7000	3000	0	0.1	2	10	1000
开始最大的搅拌	10000	7000	3000	0	0.1	2	20	5000
开始测量户外的空气	25000	10000	5000	0	0.8	4	10	10

　　Yeganeh 等表征了在生产碳基纳米材料过程中,大气中颗粒物的浓度,例如商业化的纳米技术设备生产富勒烯和碳纳米管[30]。他们在设备里面的三个地方测量细颗粒($PM_{2.5}$)的质量浓度、小于微米级别的尺寸分布、光电离电势(碳基纳米粒子的一个指标),包括在生产纳米材料的通风橱中,在通风橱外和通风橱后。一共评估了三个阶段的活动:电弧反应、清扫(即回收)、抽真空,然后比较室外的测量数据。通过比较室内和室外 $PM_{2.5}$ 的平均值和粒子计数浓度没有明显的差异。然而,大多短时间 $PM_{2.5}$ 和粒子计数浓度的增加与纳米材料的物理处理和其他生产活动相关(包括钻孔、切割石墨和金属)。在许多情况下,小于 100 nm 颗粒数量的增加在总数浓度增加中占有很大的比例。在电弧反应期时的工作环境中,检测到的数量浓度(14~673 nm)大约为 30~50000 颗粒/cm³。600000 颗粒/cm³ 的峰值主要是由于其他生产活动所造成。第二天检测到的一个较小的峰值(80000 颗粒/cm³)主要是因为进行了清扫。$PM_{2.5}$ 质量浓度范围为 50~125 μg/m³,看起来和活动的变化相关。基于在这项研究的测量中,设备中的工程控制能有效地降低纳米材料的释放暴露。

　　总之,只有两项研究被确定为与富勒烯生产活动中的职业暴露相关。一系列的方法和测量指标(颗粒数量和质量浓度)被尝试用于量化暴露情况,这两项研究显示了一些颗粒释放升高的证据。

3.3.4　二氧化钛纳米颗粒暴露及其风险评估

纳米二氧化钛（TiO_2），亦称纳米钛白粉，其外观为白色疏松粉末，具有抗紫外线、抗菌、自洁净、抗老化功效，可用于化妆品、功能纤维、塑料、油墨、涂料、油漆、精细陶瓷等领域。随着纳米 TiO_2 在工业和日常生活中的广泛应用，有必要对其职业暴露风险进行评估。

1. 暴露风险

很多研究测量的细二氧化钛释放的数据包括所有粉尘的总量，未区分可吸入组分的含量。美国的二氧化钛生产厂家曾经检测过工厂空气中的粉尘总量，超过了 10 mg/m³（IARC，1989 年），这些工厂同一时期更多的监测数据表明，在很多的工作过程中总可吸入粉尘浓度低于 3 mg/m³（中位值为 1.1 mg/m³）。细二氧化钛粒径尺寸约 0.1～0.4 μm，所以可吸入的二氧化钛颗粒占粉尘总量比例很大。1999 年针对欧洲 8 个生产细二氧化钛工厂的空气二氧化钛浓度进行了对比研究，他们检测的二氧化钛浓度范围从 0.1～5.99 mg/m³（工厂测量的最高浓度）到 0.1～0.67 mg/m³（工厂测量的最低浓度）[43]。无论是美国还是欧洲的相关研究都发现包装和粉碎操作以及机器进行维护时二氧化钛的浓度最高[44]。NIOSH 健康危害评估的结果指出，使用含有二氧化钛粉末的涂料进行涂刷操作，空气中可吸入的二氧化钛浓度范围是 0.01～1.0 mg/m³（9 个样品）（NIOSH，2009 年）。TEM 分析空气样品，结果发现 42.4% 的二氧化钛颗粒直径小于 0.1 μm。二氧化钛生产设备附近的可吸入颗粒物的浓度高达 0.14 mg/m³，TEM 结果发现大多数颗粒物的粒径范围是 25～100 nm[45]。

2. 暴露评估策略

二氧化钛生产场所现场暴露评估存在一定的复杂性，一方面需要关注悬浮颗粒在空气中的尺寸分布，可能存在细或超细颗粒；另一方面，大气中已有颗粒成分可能会干扰检测结果。二氧化钛初步风险评估应该用疏水膜收集样品（如 NIOSH 方法 0600），同时用一个混合纤维素酯过滤器（MCEF）收集粉尘样品，如果二氧化钛可呼吸暴露浓度（方法 0600 检测）小于 0.3 mg/m³，则不需要采取进一步评价工作。如果暴露浓度超过 0.3 mg/m³，就需要其他的表征方法确定二氧化钛颗粒的大小和比例以及是否有其他的外来物质。作为辅助方法，可使用 TEM 对平行收集在 MCEF 上的样品进行尺寸分析，确定颗粒尺寸以及细（>0.1 μm）和超细（<0.1 μm）二氧化钛的比例。同时还可以与能谱仪和能量损失谱联用分析颗粒物的种类（如二氧化钛）。一旦确定了二氧化钛的百分比（以颗粒尺寸划分），可以进行质量浓度的调整（按照方法 0600 来确定）以评估暴露的二氧化钛中细、超细颗

粒物或是两者的混合物是否超过 NIOSH 制定的允许暴露限值。为了使今后 TEM 分析所收集的样品最小化,可使用 NIOSH 方法 7300 或其他等效方法来确定二氧化钛的数量。当使用 NIOSH 方法 7300 时,需采取措施(即用硫酸或氢氟酸进行预处理)以确保样品的完全溶解和二氧化钛的回收率。用方法 7300 或者其他等效方法获得的结果,应该与可吸入组分的质量浓度共同确定二氧化钛浓度相对百分比。后续工作场所的暴露评估,其样品的收集分析方法推荐使用 NIOSH 方法 0600 和 7300(或等效的方法),以确保空气中的二氧化钛浓度不会随着时间的变化而变化。

3. 工作场所 TiO_2 的暴露控制

由于细二氧化钛广泛的商业用途,在许多工作场所可能存在职业暴露的情况。然而,有关二氧化钛在大气中的浓度和可能在工作场所发生暴露的数据却极为缺乏。很多报道中提到的细二氧化钛释放的数据其实都是所有粉尘的总量,而不是可呼入组分的数据。要控制工作场所二氧化钛的暴露,首先应该通过使用工程控制的手段来完成。虽然有限的数据显示存在二氧化钛的职业暴露情况,但是可以通过使用各种标准的控制技术来减少暴露风险。控制空气传播危害的标准工业卫生实践包括工程控制、工作实践、行政程序和个人防护设备。例如工程控制包括工艺改造和使用一个工业通风系统以减少工人空气传播的暴露(ACGIH,2001 年)。一般情况下,源头隔离(即从工人隔离源头的产生)和局部排气通风系统是首选的方法,防止工人暴露于气溶胶中。利用通风系统隔离暴露源和工人的常规工程控制技术,应该可以有效地降低细和超细二氧化钛的空气暴露(包括人工纳米尺度)。通风系统应配备高效微粒空气过滤器,用以除掉 99.97% 的直径为 300 nm 的颗粒。粒径小于 200 nm 的颗粒可通过扩散被收集在薄膜上,而粒径大于 800 nm 的颗粒通过压紧和拦截的作用沉积下来。通风系统必须正确设计、测试和常规维护以提供最高的工作效率。当发现工程控制和常规措施不能降低二氧化钛对工人的暴露时,那么就需要实施佩戴防尘口罩的措施。OSHA 呼吸防护标准(29 CFR 1910.134)提出了无论是自愿还是必须,都要使用防尘口罩的内容,所有标准化的内容都应被严格遵循。OSHA 呼吸防护标准的主要内容包括:①对工人戴着防尘口罩时的工作能力评估;②定期人员培训;③定期环境监测;④防尘口罩防护功能测试;⑤防尘口罩的维护、检验、清洁和保存。这项工作应该定期评估,由项目的负责人来选择防尘口罩,其对工作场所和每种防尘口罩的缺陷应有着渊博的知识。NIOSH 在他们的官方网站上提供了如何选择一个合适的防尘口罩的指导教程(http://www.cdc.gov/niosh/docs/2005-100/de-fault.html)。选择口罩时应该合理地考虑预期的暴露浓度,其他潜在的暴露和工作任务情况。对于大多数工作任务包括二氧化钛暴露,通过正确的合理测试,表明半面罩微粒防尘口罩比单一的

REL 能提供 10 倍的防护作用。防尘口罩项目的管理者基于二氧化钛颗粒的尺寸和特征,应该考虑到可能会发生滤膜上颗粒超载的情况,从而合理选择合适的滤膜和确定滤膜更换的时间。N95 型防尘口罩的过滤性能研究发现,对于 40 nm 的粒子平均穿透水平范围在 1.4%～5.2%,这表明 N95 型可以高效地捕捉空气中传播的超细二氧化钛颗粒[46,47]。雇主应该为工作场所中,对可能暴露在二氧化钛中的工人建立职业卫生监测项目。职业卫生监测项目包括风险监测(风险和承受风险的评估)和医疗监测,这是一个有效的职业安全与健康项目中重要的组成部分。项目的一个重要目标是为了预防疾病,系统地收集并分析暴露和健康的数据。对于工作场所中暴露在超细或人工纳米级二氧化钛条件下,NIOSH 发布了临时的指导步骤,采取措施尽量减少暴露的风险,建议医疗监测和筛查,这些都可用于建立合适的职业卫生监测项目。

3.3.5 纳米复合材料加工过程纳米颗粒暴露及其风险评估

术语"加工"(Matching)是指通过某种机械加工工具将一个工件的形状改变的过程,同时需要考虑加工的目的,尤其是指那些制造某一产品或通过重复性步骤,统一制造形成相同性状批量产品的过程。复合材料是指用两种或两种以上,具有明显不同物理或化学性质的材料加工形成的材料,这些材料在所形成的工件中,从宏观或微观水平上仍保持相互独立。

目前关于研究和制造消费品中使用的新型复合材料的功能信息相当的宽泛,Kumar 等调研总结了材料性质与相关产品设计之间的关系[48]。表 3.7 汇总了加工复合材料以及将纳米材料作为表面修饰材料的信息,大多用于聚合复合材料片层结构或包裹层结构中。这些参考文献中涉及的材料大多与不同的市场应用相关,这是因为一部分研究是由公司主导开展的,而研究型实验室通常使用商业化的加工件评估其安全性。

表 3.7 加工操作研究中所涉及的复合材料和包覆材料总结

纳米-复合材料	纳米-物质	参考文献
[碳纤维+CNT]环氧树脂复合	CNT	[20]
碳管包覆氧化铝基底片层,环氧树脂基质	CNT	[41]
环氧树脂包覆的碳纳米纤维	碳纳米纤维	[49]
碳纳米纤维复合物	碳纳米纤维	[49,50]
环氧树脂包覆的碳纳米纤维/碳纳米纤维片层	碳纳米纤维	[50]
水泥砂浆+CNT	CNT	[51]
聚酰胺+SiO_2 NPs	SiO_2 纳米填料,SiO_2 微粉	[51]
聚丙烯+CNT	CNT (Nanocyl NC7000)	[51]

续表

纳米-复合材料	纳米-物质	参考文献
水泥砂浆＋水化硅酸钙(CSH)	水化硅酸钙填料(纳米颗粒)	[51]
聚酰胺＋纳米黏土	黏土纳米填料	[52]
聚甲基丙烯酸甲酯＋Cu NPs	Cu NPs	[53]
聚碳酸酯,CNT-增强	CNT	[53]
聚甲基丙烯酸甲酯,CNT-增强	CNT	[54,55]
环氧基树脂,CNT-增强	CNT	[56,57]
热塑聚氨酯＋CNT	CNT (Nanocyl NC7000)	[58]
混凝土＋煅制氧化硅(Emaco Nano-Crete R4,BASF)	煅制氧化硅 (Evonik)	[59]
建筑涂料(BASF Acronal LR 8976)＋ZnO NPs	ZnO NPs 分散剂:NANOBYK-3820	[60]
清漆,Desmolux U100＋ZnO NPs	ZnO NPs: LP-X20878	[60]
聚氨酯(PU)包覆(2 种成分)＋ZnO NPs	ZnO NPs:LP-X 21217	[60,61]
建筑涂料(BASF Acronal LR 8976)＋Fe_2O_3 NPs	Fe_2O_3 NPs	[61]
紫外光硬敷层＋SiO_2	纳米 SiO_2	[62]
丙烯涂料＋TiO_2(锐钛型)	TiO_2:UV Titan	[62]
丙烯涂料＋炭黑	Flammrüss 101	[62]
户外丙烯涂料＋SiO_2	纳米 SiO_2	[62]

1. 影响测量结果的主要因素

Jordan 指出小颗粒具有彼此黏附或吸附到固体表面倾向的特性,并且这种倾向将随着颗粒变小而增大[63]。Hwang 等研究了从半导体表面移除颗粒的方法,发现当颗粒大小减小到 20~50 nm,或最后减小到 10 nm 时,颗粒移除工作变得越来越困难,吸附强度大到当用含氩气流的 30000 Torr(4 MPa)的高压氦气都不能完全清除所黏附颗粒[64]。对于复合材料,有必要先考虑基质材料与纳米颗粒界面上的吸附力情况,已有利用原子力显微镜悬臂拉扯出单根 CNT 进行测量拉伸强度的报道[65,66],根据所用基质材料的不同,所测量到的界面剪切力从几兆帕到几百兆帕不等,强度大致相当于涤纶长丝,但明显要小于单根 CNT 的强度,其可达 10000 MPa,当 CNT 嵌入基质中被拉伸出来时所需要的力明显要远小于达到使其断裂的强度所需要的拉伸力。

复合新材料在飞机配套产品制造及用于加工超硬耐磨损材料的高级专业加工设备领域有着很好的应用,复合材料的成分可以是有机材料(产品件)或无机材料(加工工具),从而在加工过程产生气溶胶颗粒,可能是来源于工件或加工工具本身,或两者都有。另外一些加工技术本身没有加工工具与工件的直接接触,比如电加工过程中的电火花加工(EDM)[67,68],使用激光加工时,其中一种是利用紫外光波脉冲原理[69],还有使用飞秒超短波原理的[70],这些操作均通过形成等离子体的形式将材料加工去除掉,通常在此过程中等离子体中会凝集化合物而会形成大量的超微颗粒物,同样,此原理过程可以反向应用,比如用激光烧蚀法合成单壁碳纳米管就是如此[71]。

人们对按照颗粒物粒径大小分级给出的结果感兴趣,是因为可以表明纳米材料是单颗粒释放还是以形成团聚物的形式,而通常存在一个超细颗粒物背景干扰的问题。背景干扰的产生是现代社会广泛存在的机械化背景导致的,包括内燃机的尾气或电动机电圈释出的铜纳米颗粒。一些作者将高水平的超细颗粒物背景归咎于电动机的释放[51,72,73]。一些电动机如铜整流器上有碳刷滑动类型的,更容易产生大量的超细颗粒物[74,75]。在纳米实验室或制造工厂中生产含有纳米材料产品时也可能会产生交叉污染问题。从高温到低温的冷凝过程通常会形成圆形颗粒物团聚(均一凝结核条件),他们可以通过电镜和物理化学分析方法进行鉴定。团聚情况的存在使结果阐释过程更加困难费时,因为现在快速检测且价格较低的常用仪器,不能在颗粒物计数时去除背景颗粒物。然而,仍然可以通过测定并剔除典型背景颗粒物分布数据,从而获得所检测纳米材料特异释放的信息;或者通过隔离外界背景环境进行检测实现,后者通常使用隔离装置并补充过滤掉颗粒物的空气,或者在洁净间内进行,再或防尘罩内进行。McGarry 等的文章中详细描述了如何剔除纳米释放过程中背景颗粒物的影响[75]。

众所周知,固体超微颗粒物一般存在很强的团聚倾向并形成多孔的形态,而不是规则圆形。另外,有着大量生产纳米纤维如碳管的情况,这类物质的存在形态主要体现在其二次形态,而不是纳米纤维基本的长度和直径。随着碳管或无机管状类物质如氮化硼纳米管状材料的出现,气溶胶科学就遇到了一个问题,即纤维容易形成缠结或球形结构,与其基本的长度和直径形状相比,这些高长径比物质在气流环境下所体现的缠结或球形结构更具有代表性意义。这些形状决定着纳米材料在空气中的状态,决定着它们是如何进肺的,吸入后又是如何沉积的。在通过迁移率测定时,二次形态决定着纳米材料的空气动力学大小,就必须考虑这些纤维丝状构成的结构极度蓬松,因此密度仅为相同大小材料密度的很小的部分。类似于气凝胶颗粒,纳米材料的实际大小与空气动力学大小差异很大,这是因为这两个参数是根据较高密度固体乳胶球进行匹配校准的。

纳米纤维类物质的二次形态差异很大,取决于其形成的环境。例如,当用超声分散碳纳米管时,碳纳米管可以随着气溶胶中的液滴迁移,碳纳米管的二次形态就取决于气化液滴的大小。当如果碳纳米管嵌入聚合物基质中时,基质表面随着紫外线照射降解,贴近表面的碳纳米管就会暴露于空气中,这种情况下,二次形态就由碳纳米管在基质中的嵌入情况所决定。从而,很难通过纳米纤维本身的几何尺寸如纤维长度和直径来定义其空气释放性状,而应当考虑其二次形态,并需要注意它们是可以变化成不同形状的。

2. 调研的加工过程种类

调研的加工过程种类包括常规加工像磨、砂光、锯切、车削、铣削,总结在表3.8中,还包括更多新型的但越来越重要的过程,像在加工超硬材料和复合材料时使用的电火花加工(EDM)、搅拌摩擦焊(FSW)和超短脉冲激光切割加工技术。聚焦离子束(FIB)铣削技术通常不作为"加工"过程,但这一观点可能会随着纳米尺度上的精度操作发展而得以改变。同样存在一些属于受控实验特定设定的过程,专门用于检测颗粒释放,模拟在消费产品在使用时的效应情况,如磨损测试或光照暴露(紫外线照射仓)。磨损测试起初是用于测定固形物或织物的耐久性的,现在用于检测使用过程中的颗粒释放情况,紫外线照射仓照射可用于模拟日光照射,Hsu等进行的一项研究是同时考察了磨损(橡胶刀片刮板)、照射(紫外灯)及风(风扇)同时作用的效应[31]。

表 3.8　加工过程与被加工材料总结表[76]

加工	过程	纳米-材料(纳米物质)	参考文献
磨损	砂纸板	• 聚酰胺+SiO_2 NP	[51]
		• 聚丙烯+CNT	
		• 水泥+CNT	
		• 水泥+CSH	
		• 热塑性聚氨酯+CNT	[58]
	Taber 旋转	• 聚酰胺+SiO_2 NP	[51]
		• 聚丙烯+CNT	
		• 水泥+CNT	
		• 水泥+CSH	
		• 热塑性聚氨酯+CNT	[58]
		• 聚氨酯+ZnO	[60]
		• 清漆+ZnO	
		• 建筑包覆+ZnO	
	美国泰伯尔,一次性	• 环氧基树脂+CNT	[57]
		• 聚甲基丙烯酸甲酯+Cu NP	[53]
		• 聚碳酸酯+CNT	
		• 聚对苯二甲酸乙二醇酯织物+聚氯乙烯包覆+纳米黏土	[77]

续表

加工	过程	纳米-材料(纳米物质)	参考文献
切割	带锯	• (非纳米级碳纤维+CNT) 环氧树脂 • (氧化铝纤维+CNT) 环氧树脂	[20]
	圆盘锯 (湿法)	• (非纳米级碳纤维+CNT) 环氧树脂 • (氧化铝纤维+CNT) 环氧树脂	[20]
		• 碳纳米纤维复合料	[49,50]
	磨	• 铝合金	[78]
		非 (Li-Ti-MO)	[33]
钻	水泥钻	• 纳米克里特水泥(煅制氧化硅)	[72]
	长绞钻 (flute-reamer)	• 双马来酰亚胺/ 石墨烯(硬质合金)	[79]
	多晶 钻石钻	• 双马来酰亚胺/ 石墨烯	[79]
	研磨钻	• (非纳米级碳纤维+CNT) 环氧树脂	[80]
		• (氧化铝纤维+CNT) 环氧树脂	[80]
电火花	钨电流	• 聚甲基丙烯酸甲酯+CNT	[54,55]
摩擦搅 拌焊	铣削	• 铝合金	[81]
研磨	微量研磨机	• 热喷涂 (碳化钨-12Co；Al_2O_3-13TiO_2)	[82]
	研磨机	• 环氧树脂-碳纳米纤维航天复合材料	[50]
		• 花岗岩	[83]
		• 陶瓷黏土	
		• 硬木	
激光	飞秒级	无(Ag NP)	[84]
		无	[69]
纳米磨	聚焦离子束	• 聚甲基丙烯酸甲酯+CNT	[85]
打磨	手工	• 环氧树脂+CNT	[56]
		• 环氧树脂-碳纳米纤维内含料/碳纳米纤维 片层	[50]
	微型	• 聚氨酯-ZnO	[61]
		• AC-ZnO	
		• AC-Fe_2O_3	

续表

加工	过程	纳米-材料(纳米物质)	参考文献
	轨道	• 聚醋酸乙烯酯涂料＋TiO₂	[73,86]
		• 亚克力涂料＋TiO₂	[86]
		• 亚克力涂料＋CB	
		• 紫外硬膜＋SiO₂	
	皮带	• 环氧树脂-碳纳米纤维航天复合材料	[50]
旋转式	车床	• 铝合金,低碳钢,高强度钢(工具:金属陶瓷)	[87,88]
		• 无（工具：Si₃N₄晶须；TiN NP）	[89]
	数控车床	• 碳纤维加强复合材料（工具：碳化钨；TiC）	[90]
气候	紫外照射	• 聚酰胺＋SiO₂ NP	[51]
		• 聚丙烯＋CNT	
		• 水泥＋CNT	
		• 水泥＋CSH	
		• 热塑性聚氨酯＋CNT	[58]
		• 环氧树脂＋SiO₂	[91]
		• 环氧树脂＋MWCNT	
		光催化涂料＋TiO₂	[31]

表 3.9 给出了测量过程中释放出的颗粒物。

表 3.9　所释放颗粒物汇总表[76]

加工过程 （工具）	颗粒源(纳米器件)	采样器:暴露说明	文献
打磨 （砂纸）	复合材料： • PA＋SiO₂ NP（SiO₂） • POM＋CNT（CNT） • 水泥＋CNT（CNT） • 水泥＋CSH（CSH）	产生粉尘的直径大小 （10～80 μm）. • 仅 POM： ＞400 nm • POM＋CNT： ＞700 nm • CEM＋CNT： ＞130 nm	[51]
打磨 （Taber 旋转打磨）	• 环氧树脂＋CNT(CNT)	四种模式宽范围粒径谱仪： 326～415 nm;≈680 nm;≈1200 nm; 2300～2400nm 发现基质颗粒,CNT 突出形态,游离及聚合形态的颗粒	[57]

续表

加工过程 （工具）	颗粒源(纳米器件)	采样器:暴露说明	文献
打磨 (Taber 线 性打磨)	• PET 纤维 　＋PVC 涂层 　＋纳米黏土	峰值处的颗粒直径: • PET: 80 nm • PET＋PVC: 80 nm • PET＋PVC＋纳米黏土: 50 nm	[77]
	复合材料 • PMMA＋Cu NP (Cu) • Polycarb＋CNT (CNT)	PC-CNT 电镜没发现纳米颗粒及碳管 PMMA-Cu:微米级颗粒发现 Cu,且 Cu 颗粒几乎都是与基质分开的	[53]
切割 (带锯)	复合材料 • [CF＋CNT] 环氧树脂 • [铝纤维＋CNT]环氧树脂 (CNT)	• 大量 10～20 nm 颗粒(圆形,团聚) • 直径 30 nm～6 μm 纤维成分,有部分 直径 300 nm 的纤维有 10 μm 长,无 游离的 CNTs	[20]
切割(湿 法,钻石, 圆锯)	复合材料 • 环氧树脂包覆的 CNF (CNF) • CNF 复合料材(CNF)	• 直径 30～200 nm • 湿法切割主要直径 400 nm • 碳纳米纤维直径约 500 nm	[49]
	• 环氧树脂-CNF 太空复合材料	• 基质成分 • 大量碳纳米纤维,有游离碳纳米纤维 成分 • 团聚碳纳米纤维	[50]
钻孔	复合材料 • [CF＋CNT]环氧树脂(CNT) • [铝纤维＋CNT] 环氧树脂(CNT)	团聚的可呼入颗粒 • 团聚的碳管 • <10 nm 部分是圆形颗粒,白烟下的 沉积物	[80]
钻孔 (手持)	器件: 水泥＋SiO_2 添加(SiO_2)	颗粒平均直径 37～51 nm;大小在 19～ 300 nm	[72]
研磨 (石质磨盘)	• 环氧树脂-CNF 太空复合材料	• 基质材料成分 • 高浓度超细颗粒,很少部分是 CNT	[50]
打磨 (手工)	复合材料: • CNT-环氧树脂(CNT)	• 电镜下大颗粒＞300 nm 有聚合状态 的 CNT • 无游离 CNT	[56]
	• 环氧树脂-CNF 复合材料/ CNF 巴克纸片基	有碳纳米纤维存在	[50]

续表

加工过程 （工具）	颗粒源（纳米器件）	采样器:暴露说明	文献
打磨 （小型 打磨机）	聚氨酯（PU）或 建筑涂料（AC）： • PU-ZnO（ZnO） • AC-ZnO（ZnO） • AC-Fe$_2$O$_3$（Fe$_2$O$_3$）	SEM 下主要是直径＞20 μm	[92]
打磨 （带形）	• 环氧树脂-CNF 太空复合材料	• 主要是基质成分 • 可以检测到 CNF，但无游离 CNF • 有团聚圆形碳纳米颗粒成分	[50]

　　干燥切割含有多壁碳管复合物时明显产生大量纳米或超细颗粒物，比如在不同材料复合物中（碳纳米管-碳材料，碳纳米管-矾土材料，对照），同时可以产生亚微米长度纳米直径的纤维和更大些的可吸入纤维，最小的在透射电镜下看到的独立纳米纤维大约 30 nm 直径，几百纳米长，明显是来源于复合材料中的碳纳米管纤维，没有多壁碳管释放出来的证据[20]。

　　对于复合多壁碳管的材料，钻孔[80]与切割[20]在大小分布、纤维成分浓度及颗粒形态上有不同，另外钻孔时在电镜下发现有碳纳米管成分的聚合成分。在研究加工复合材料时，电镜发现有碳纳米管成分，但没发现自由释放出的碳纳米管[56]，另外一项研究报告显示纳米颗粒有释放，但没有发现碳纳米管释放出来[53]。在 13 项研究加工纳米纤维的成果中，12 项显示电镜可以看到释放出的纳米纤维成分[50]，大部分是非聚合存在的纳米纤维，一小部分呈现输送聚合的纳米纤维。总结如下，加工含纳米颗粒的复合材料时可以发现下面种类的颗粒释放：

　　• 纳米材料嵌入所用基质成分颗粒。

　　• 可以发现明显的颗粒释放，主要来自于基质成分，但是期间释放出的纳米颗粒有来自于材料中的纳米材料成分。

　　• 仅在一项摩擦操作研究中发现有释放出来的游离碳纳米管，其他加工碳纳米管复合材料的研究没有发现类似情况[57]。一项研究发现加工碳纳米管纤维复合材料时有碳纳米管纤维的释放[50]。

　　• 在钻孔和摩擦操作中发现团聚的碳纳米管情况[57]。

　　• 纳米成分从多聚纳米颗粒中凸显出来有很多例证，包括环氧树脂碳纳米管复合[56]，摆设建筑涂料[60]或聚氨酯中[92]的氧化锌纳米颗粒，以及聚甲基丙烯酸甲酯中的铜纳米颗粒[53]。

　　总体结论是：①有纳米成分复合的材料与无纳米成分复合的材料相比，在线监测的颗粒释放水平间没有明显区别。②高能加工过程相比低能过程产生明显更多的颗粒释放,产生更高的气溶胶质量浓度。③湿法加工与干燥加工相比释放水平明显低得多,见文献[20,80]。然而,湿法锯切仍然产生大量的颗粒释放情况[50]。④大量因素可影响释放程度的预测,因此,现在为止仍缺少足够的数据能对不同材料释放水平下结论。⑤所释放纳米颗粒物是混合物包括基质颗粒及复合材料纳米成分。⑥对于暴露控制,工程控制可以减少或防止机械加工过程中的工人暴露,一些证据显示控制及设计对于防止暴露情况发生至关重要。

第4章　纳米颗粒暴露监测流程及相关仪器

4.1　纳米颗粒呼吸暴露监测要点

4.1.1　概述

纳米颗粒暴露监测是一项巨大的挑战,其任务包括如何与背景颗粒进行区分,仪器选择,收集、分析颗粒尺寸及其分布特征,空间及时间变化规律,甚至包括如何测量分析高长径比的纳米颗粒等。

4.1.2　区分释放的颗粒物与背景颗粒物

典型的城市环境空气中每立方厘米大致含有 10000～40000 个颗粒物,它们来源于多种释放途径,包括工业污染、交通及颗粒物输运扩散等。这些背景颗粒的粒径通常小于 1000 nm,并且大多介于 10～300 nm,给生产场所中纳米颗粒的释放监测工作造成一定的困难。

一般可以采用三种方法克服背景颗粒物的影响,这些方法可以单独或者联合使用。第一种是按时间的顺序分开进行监测,同时记录发生事件,例如对预热反应器的运作记录,从而合理地建立事件与监测数据之间的关联。第二种是用相同仪器平行监测无颗粒释放的位置情况,通常称为"远端"监测,例如远离实验室或生产场所的位置。监测时需要特别注意,所监测的背景位置不能有类似释放源或其他颗粒的释放。第三种是收集气溶胶颗粒,用于离线分析,从而验证所监测到的颗粒释放峰值是所监测的纳米颗粒。离线分析技术通常包括含量分析(如元素或杂质含量)和形态分析,如扫描、透射电镜及能谱分析等。

在应用这些方法的过程中,应注意实验条件要求,比如监测时间不同导致远端背景监测时条件不一致,从而造成数据错误。联合应用上述方法效果会更好,可对工作场所中是否存在某种纳米颗粒释放进行定性判断,比如判定监测位置与远端位置颗粒监测数值的比率(比如设定比值 1.05 作为判定阈值),监测到的浓度与尺寸分布的变化结果是否与记录事件相吻合,以及近端与远端所监测颗粒化学成分特征是否与预期一致。但这些监测方法本身具有一定的局限性,比如动态响应时间、监测精度及测量的不确定性,导致监测时不一定能够根据变化比例监测到颗粒释放的显著变化,并且现有的监测方法的精度大多不高。

4.1.3　颗粒物粒径检测

　　颗粒物粒径及其分布特征是颗粒物暴露监测的重要参数,通常可以使用多种仪器进行测量。实验室产生的气溶胶颗粒尺寸分布并不总是呈现一定的规律,通常更为复杂,有时呈现双峰分布,尺寸较小的峰通常表示颗粒本身,而尺寸较大的峰可能是颗粒自身聚集/团聚或与背景颗粒聚集/团聚形成的峰,因此,不能简单地使用平均粒径或几何平均数来描述。

　　扫描电迁移率粒径谱仪(Scanning Mobility Particle Sizer/Stepped Mobility Particle Sizer, SMPS)和快速电迁移率粒径谱仪(Fast Mobility Particle Sizer, FMPS)能够给出详细的颗粒尺寸分布数据。这些数据可以通过多种形式进行分析,最常用的是监测整个粒径谱分布,尤其适用于一次事件或一次变化的分析,例如对背景进行测量,或者对比背景颗粒与释放的颗粒。但是,粒径谱数据比较难以描述,比如双峰分布不能用几何平均数及变异系数来进行对比描述。

　　另一种替代方法是计算颗粒总数,但这种方式不具备尺寸分布信息,大大降低了测量数据的意义。一些研究人员将粒径分布信息进行分段汇总,如<10 nm,<100 nm ,<1000 nm 等,并与时间关联,从而将颗粒释放情况与背景进行区分或描述颗粒动力学形成过程[20,29],此种方法对于描述气溶胶分布随时间改变十分有效。

4.1.4　最大可检测颗粒尺寸上限

　　劳动防护暴露界定了与颗粒尺寸相关的健康安全阈值标准[27]。合成或使用纳米材料的工作场所中气溶胶颗粒分布范围很广,在表征纳米材料过程中需要界定最大颗粒的尺寸,通常排除粒径大于 100 nm 的颗粒。已有研究表明释放的颗粒很少以单一纳米颗粒形式存在,通常以聚集/团聚或与背景颗粒聚集/团聚的形式存在。大多数研究从最大化获得数据的角度出发,研究整个颗粒尺寸分布谱,而不是截取其中某一段进行分析。通常认为聚集/团聚是纳米材料导致,从毒理学角度出发,需要在风险评估时考虑到这些大的聚集/团聚颗粒的解聚及析出过程。

　　很多仪器具有最大可检测颗粒限值,如凝聚核粒子计数器(CPC)入口有撞击器可去掉过大的颗粒,最大颗粒限值是 1 μm。过大的颗粒会降低检测效率,入口撞击器可用于保护仪器检测系统。当考虑数量浓度这一参数时,需要进行合理的标准化,否则,两台不同最大限值的仪器将给出不同的监测结果。另外,一些研究人员建议使用可吸入颗粒作为测量上限,这样可以将劳动防护暴露与生物效应联系起来[27]。

4.1.5　颗粒物释放的时空变化

工作环境中接近释放源处的气溶胶浓度较高,随着距离的变化而变化。Demou 等报道了在不同测试情况下也存在或高或低的变化,他们监测了纳米颗粒释放到无颗粒物和有颗粒物的环境,发现纳米颗粒能快速与背景气溶胶团聚进而被湮没掉[32]。

现场监测中存在时间与空间上的高变异性,这就使个人剂量监测变得十分重要,例如在工人呼吸区利用相关仪器进行测量。已有研究显示,个人暴露监测通常要比针对环境的暴露监测所测得的数值更高,这通常是由于与静态的环境监测仪器相比,工人通常更接近到释放源位置,同时,释放活动通常由工人的活动引起的,远离释放源位置的暴露水平显著降低。这与纳米颗粒的传输、团聚及清除率明显相关。

4.1.6　测量参数

在测量纳米颗粒暴露的过程中,主要有三个参数:①质量浓度(mg/m^3);②数量浓度(个$/m^3$);③表面积浓度(m^2/m^3)。在不同环境下应当使用不同的测量检测参数,遵循的原则是选择的参数要与潜在健康危害尽量直接相关。通常需要同时检测这三个参数才能够更好地进行影响评价。

这三个参数的测量都可以用特定的仪器获得,对于质量浓度,一个重要的问题是缺乏针对纳米颗粒进行监测的灵敏仪器,而颗粒数量浓度监测相比要灵敏的多,然而仅仅监测颗粒数量浓度将很可能对于暴露评估造成误导。在所有的数量浓度监测中,需要关注不同仪器的检测限以进行合理的数据分析,实时监测纳米颗粒表面积技术上是可行的,但这种类型的仪器尚不多见。所有监测结果都需要结合仪器特点进行详细分析,同时还需要考虑颗粒携带的电荷、化学组分、聚集/团聚状态(特别是颗粒表面积及所组成颗粒的总表面积)以及颗粒形状。

最理想的监测参数,应该是与所涉及的健康效应直接相关,能够容易监测,同时在动态变化范围内得到灵敏有效的监测结果。

4.1.7　高长径比的纳米颗粒暴露评估

WHO 对可吸入纤维成分定义为纤维长度大于 5×10^{-6} m (5000 nm),宽度(直径)小于 3×10^{-6} m (3000 nm),长径比大于 3:1。对于纤维类气溶胶通常监测其数量浓度,如在光镜下进行计数,并有效计算成束及交错组成的纤维,最后统计数量浓度。该方法适用于高长径比的纳米颗粒暴露评价(BSI 6699-2:2007;BSI,2007 年)。

评估碳纳米管材料时,会出现一些问题,尽管光镜可以看到成束的碳纳米管,但却不能监测到单根的碳纳米管,而高倍电子显微镜比如 SEM/TEM 将会使计数时间大大延长。由于光镜观察不到单根碳纳米管,这样得到的数据将大大低估了碳纳米管纤维的数量浓度,而电镜观察同样的样本所统计的数量浓度将比光镜大。这样,很难与光镜下设定的纤维数量阈值进行比对评价。

4.2 纳米颗粒现场监测仪器介绍

4.2.1 撞击分级采样器

撞击分级采样器是气溶胶采样方法之一,它可以提供与粒径分布相对应的质量分布。仪器由一系列的收集器组成,每一层都有相应的切割头,用于收集特定粒径的气溶胶样品。每一级收集的颗粒物将进行进一步分析,例如,X 衍射可以提供晶体结构信息,电感耦合等离子体质谱(ICP-MS)提供关于纳米颗粒的化学成分信息。

4.2.2 锥形元件振荡微量天平

锥形元件振荡微量天平(Tapered Element Oscillating Microbalance,TEOM)能够自动监测气溶胶质量浓度,它是目前为止唯一一类单一操作分析大量气溶胶样品的仪器,先将气溶胶收集到采样膜上再进行沉积质量的测量,气溶胶的收集可以观察振动频率的变化,这种变化与收集到的颗粒物的质量呈正相关(实际是频率平方的倒数),TEOM 是环境空气质量监测站的标准监测仪器。PM_{10}、$PM_{2.5}$ 和 PM_1 选择器的安装能够采集环境中气溶胶被空气动力学切割成直径 10 μm、2.5 μm 或 1 μm 的样品。欧洲安全与健康机构推荐的这些选择器符合环保标准,但不同于在工业卫生领域收集的气溶胶数据,特别是可吸入部分(切割粒径 4 μm)的颗粒物。此外,TEOM 仪器的重量和尺寸意味着只可以用于静态环境采样,不能用于动态采样。

4.2.3 扫描电迁移率粒径谱仪

扫描电迁移率粒径谱仪(Scanning Mobility Particle Sizer,SMPS)用于检测颗粒物粒径分布。它是由静电迁移率分析仪(DMA)和粒子计数器(CPC)组成。DMA 可用于筛分出不同粒径的气溶胶,气溶胶被内置真空泵吸入到主机内,主机中有梯度变化的电场、电压,荷电的气溶胶在电场中受电场力的作用产生迁移现象,在鞘气的携带下向某一方向运动,并最终沉积在电场中的某一点,如果所带电荷相同,则粒径小的颗粒在电场中飞行的距离短,粒径大的颗粒在电场中飞行的距离长,通过调节电压可以实现在同一位置采集不同粒径的颗粒;内置检测器用于检测 DMA 筛分出的不同粒径的气溶胶。由内置泵将样气抽气进入仪器内部,并和仪器中的饱和蒸汽混合,混合的气体马上进入温度较低的冷凝室,由于温度突然降低,饱和蒸汽达到过饱和状态,从而产生凝结现象,使较小的气溶胶颗粒变大,便于检测器检测,从而得到气溶胶的数量浓度;内置的气溶胶中和器电离空气产生正负离子,中和气溶胶表面的多余电荷,保证空气中的气溶胶达到波尔兹曼平衡分布,达到波尔兹曼平衡分布的气溶胶进入 CPC,准确检测到气溶胶的数量浓度。SMPS 的测量范围从几纳米到微米之间。但是该仪器过大的尺寸和重量限制了其在环境监测中的使用。

4.2.4　静电低压撞击器

静电低压撞击器(Electrical Low Pressure Impactor,ELPI)自动监测颗粒物数量浓度和粒径分布,测量范围是空气动力学直径为 6 nm～10 μm 的颗粒。气溶胶颗粒进入已知电量的电晕加电机内,然后,颗粒物进入到一个具有低压若干级的电绝缘分离取样器内,根据颗粒物的空气动力学直径和其携带到取样器内并由灵敏静电计感应到的电荷,颗粒物被收集进入不同级的取样器。这种感应到的电信号与颗粒的数量浓度和尺寸直接成正比。根据颗粒尺寸与加电机的性能和采样等级的相互关系,可将检测到的电信号转化为颗粒物的粒径分布。结果是实时的采集到的颗粒物数量和粒径分布。通过关闭加电装置,可以用 ELPI 进行颗粒物电荷分布的测量。该仪器的重量、静态固定采样限制了它的使用。与传统的碰撞采样仪相同,可以对每个收集层的颗粒物进行化学分析,最后层级在纳米级范围,使得这台仪器非常具有优势。

4.2.5　粒子计数器

粒子计数器(Condensation Particle Counter,CPC,或称凝聚核计数器,Condensation Nuclei Counter,CNC)可以通过激光检测空气样品的颗粒数量浓度,光学读数最大灵敏度的颗粒直径为 100 nm,这就需要所监测颗粒粒径增大到可监测的范围内再进行测定,所以样品颗粒需通过有机溶剂或水蒸气冷凝结核,这种粒径增大方式的仪器可检测的颗粒物粒径最小是 3 nm,因此,CPC 或 CNC 检测气溶胶样品不受颗粒物粒径尺寸的限制。它们主要用于洁净间内环境污染物如粉尘等是否处于较低水平的检测,制定洁净间颗粒物标准浓度范围。此外,仪器的尺寸和重量只允许用于环境监测。

4.2.6　纳米颗粒表面积浓度监测仪

纳米颗粒表面积浓度监测仪(Nanoparticle Surface Area Monitor,NSAM)用于测量沉积在呼吸道支气管或肺泡部分的气溶胶颗粒表面积浓度。采集的气溶胶颗粒表面带电,颗粒带电数与其表面积直接相关。荷电颗粒被收集到膜上,通过检测阻抗时间确定表面积浓度。适当调节离子捕集器的参数可以直接给出在气管或肺泡区域沉积的颗粒表面积浓度。这是一个完整的监测方法,但它不能提供采集颗粒物的粒径分布情况。仪器的重量限制了它仅适用于静态环境采样。

建议纳米颗粒暴露监测的基本仪器配置如下:

(1) 手持粒子计数器(CPC)。CPC(ISO/PWI 2789:2008)检测每立方米空气颗粒总数(P/cc)。评估的最低要求是:粒径范围在 10～1000 nm(1 μm);监测范围从 0 到 100000 P/cc。

(2) 手持光学粒子计数器(OPC)。OPC (ISO 21501-4:2007, ISO/DIS 21501-1:2008)可以依据模型测量一定粒径范围的颗粒总数。最少需要以下粒径范围的评估:300～500 nm;500～1000 nm;1000～10000 nm 以及>10000 nm。

(3) 依据纳米颗粒的类型和分析项目选择适当的空气采样滤膜(如混合纤维素酯,石英纤维过滤膜等)。可以使用特别配备了 TEM 格栅的过滤器,就不必在准备滤膜前分析 TEM[36]。

(4) 空气采样泵可在高流速下采样(10 L/min 或其他流量),取决于采样时间、所需的表征方法和相应的标准(如果有可用的标准)。

(5) 热沉淀器(Thermal Precipitator,TP)将纳米颗粒物收集到硅床上,而静电沉淀器(Electro Static Precipitator,ESP)将纳米颗粒收集到 TEM 格栅上。SEM 与能谱联用可提供颗粒物形态和化学成分的信息。

(6) 采样泵流量校准仪。

4.3 纳米材料生产过程中潜在颗粒释放评估

4.3.1 释放源辨识

可通过回顾生产过程、类型、工艺流程、材料投入和排出、工作任务和工作时间来辨识释放源。通过参考资料(如 MSDS,原始材料记录)获得纳米材料生产或使用的信息,包括材料的尺寸、形状、溶解度等理化性质。一旦能够确认生产过程中存在潜在释放源,工业环境卫生学家(或其他有资格的人)可以进行如下工作:

对生产区域和流程进行现场调查,确定释放源;

确定每个操作的频率和持续时间以及用于储存材料的容器和加工设备的类型;

确定是否有排气通风措施及其运转情况。初步评估包括识别潜在的系统故障可能导致排放控制/控制系统,如管线中有无泄漏孔,密封垫片腐蚀泄漏等。

确定生产过程中可能发生的违反管理规程的操作(如产品回收或清洗时直接

打开封闭系统等违规操作)。

4.3.2 颗粒数量浓度检测

1. 背景值测量

在生产纳米材料前,检测人员(或其他有资格的人)使用 CPC 与 OPC 测定不同过程与不同区域的背景浓度。如果所测颗粒数量浓度高(数值是相对的,会随着工艺和设施的不同而不同),则需评估是否在该地区有纳米颗粒释放源。纳米颗粒有多种来源,包括真空泵、天然气供热单元、汽油/丙烷/柴油机动车、其他燃烧或产热过程(如焊接或热封)。CPC 与 OPC 可以用来检查纳米级颗粒物的释放是否来自这些过程。室外或循环空气的建筑通风系统也应该被视为一个可能的纳米级颗粒物的释放源。

颗粒物背景浓度的测量需在所考察的流程(纳米材料制造或加工结束)结束后再次进行。计算背景浓度的平均值,并用制造或加工纳米颗粒过程中的监测值减去背景值来评估释放情况。只有背景颗粒数在观测阶段自始至终保持相对稳定,并且在调查过程中颗粒的释放显著高于背景值时,这种方法才是可以接受的。在其他情况下,背景的颗粒浓度校正变得更加复杂,需要额外的在一个较长的时间周期内采样来确定排放源和背景颗粒浓度大小。这种评价方案一般适用于初始评估阶段。

2. 区域采样

一旦确定了初始背景颗粒浓度,就可以用 CPC 和 OPC 在疑似排放源(例如,打开反应器、处理产品、在通风系统潜在的泄漏点)附近位置进行空气中颗粒浓度和粒度范围的测量。对每个检测任务之前、期间和之后大气颗粒物浓度进行监测,是为了确定一些因素(如控制、人员互动、工作实施)是否影响空气颗粒物浓度。这些信息进一步与操作过程、位置及滤膜采样测量等数据关联。

4.4　区域空气采样及个人暴露空气采样

4.4.1 区域空气采样

将纳米材料生产或加工场所的空气样品收集到滤膜上,并同时用 CPC 和 OPC 检测空气中颗粒物的浓度。对滤膜进行称重、电镜观察或元素质量测定等分析,可以得到颗粒尺寸、形状、质量、化学成分等数据,例如,收集的一部分样品可进行金属检测(参考 NIOSH 方法 7303)或碳元素检测(参考 NIOSH 方法 5040),以确定纳米颗粒组成。其余样品可以参考 NIOSH 方法 7402、7404 等进行颗粒物表征。

　　收集空气样品时,要尽可能地靠近释放源,增加监测到颗粒物的概率。应依据纳米颗粒释放特征、工人操作时间等确定采样时间。如果纳米颗粒释放持续时间很短(如几分钟),则需要相对高的空气采样流量(如 10 L/min),以确保足够多的颗粒沉积至滤膜上。如果颗粒数量浓度(采用 CPC 或 OPC 测定)很高,对于 TEM或 SEM 样品表征,则需缩短采样时间以避免过度沉积干扰颗粒物表征。如果用于电镜表征,采样时间通常为 15~30 min,如果 CPC 或 OPC 显示颗粒数量浓度高,那么采样时间可缩短至 5~10 min,或者分别进行短时间和长时间的样品收集,以确保足够的样品用于电镜分析。在远离纳米颗粒释放位置处,最少应收集两个背景滤膜样品。

4.4.2　个人暴露空气采样

　　个人呼吸区(PBZ)空气样品检测可以提供工人暴露于纳米材料的可能性及暴露程度,这些工人包括协助处理纳米材料,或操作可能导致颗粒释放的相关仪器设备等人。如果 CPC 和 OPC 测量发现工人接触区域存在纳米级的颗粒物释放,那么就应该进行 PBZ 采样。PBZ 样品分析方式与区域空气样品相同,例如 TEM 和元素质量分析等。如果任务持续的时间和由此产生的潜在风险较短暂,那么样品收集需要较高的流量(如 10 L/min)。

4.4.3　其他可选采样

　　1. 空气采样

　　OPC 测量表明很大一部分(超过 50%)的颗粒尺寸超过 1000 nm,当使用个体级联碰撞器或有过滤器的呼吸采样器采样,再进行元素含量和 TEM/SEM 电镜分析,需要去除掉大颗粒物,这可能干扰结论分析。如果生产或使用二氧化钛,建议使用 NIOSH 的采样草案:对职业接触二氧化钛(Occupational Exposure to Titanium Dioxide)的健康危害评价和建议,并按照 NIOSH 方法 0600 收集监测气溶胶质量浓度数据。

　　2. 表面沾染颗粒物采样

　　人造纳米材料可能会污染设备或其他物品表面,对这些表面颗粒物的采集监测不属于常规评估,也不能提供具体尺寸信息,但可以确定是否存在表面污染情况,也可以用于评估控制措施的有效性。是否进行表面样品监测由监测人员进行确定,并取决于人们是否对这些纳米材料感兴趣,例如,为了确定灰尘中是否有量子点的表面污染,可分析收集的表面样品中是否含有量子点的化学成分。表面擦拭样品的收集按照标准预润湿基质方法,如元素分析 NIOSH 9102(NIOSH,1994年)。采集样本分析时的手套和工具应该分别销毁,避免交叉污染。

4.4.4　质量控制

为确保有效的暴露测量数据,应该按照以下质量控制步骤进行:

(1) 使用工厂校准的直读式测量分析仪器;

(2) 每次使用前校准所有粒子计数器至零点;

(3) 每天采样前后进行泵的校准;

(4) 除了对采集的样品进行分析,还需对空白对照进行分析。

标准物质(Reference Material,RM)是均一、稳定且性质明确的一类材料,可以用于不同的途径,包括质量控制、方法校准等。目前,人造纳米材料领域已经有了一些标准物质,例如,美国国家标准与技术研究院的金纳米材料(RM8011、RM8012、RM8013);欧洲委员会联合研究中心研究所的二氧化硅胶体材料(IRMM-304)。它们是球形材料,主要认证信息是尺寸和性能,因此可用于校准和仪器粒度测量的质量控制。当前缺少公认的暴露指标及检测方法,如粒径分布、数量浓度和/或表面积以及标准化测试方法,这成为标准物质生产的主要障碍。

4.4.5　数据分析

1. 粒径

由于空气中人造纳米材料的尺寸和聚集程度在样品采集时是未知的,应用直读粒子尺寸/计数仪器,可以减去背景颗粒数从而提供半定量的潜在释放评估。CPC 可提供测量每立方厘米粒子尺寸 10~1000 nm 范围的空气总数值。OPC 可以提供在以下至少四个具体的尺寸范围:300~500 nm,500~1000 nm,1000~10000 nm 以及>10000 nm 每升空气中颗粒的总数。如有必要,可以使用 CPC 和 OPC 数据共同确定纳米颗粒的数量浓度。例如,CPC 测得的颗粒浓度高,而 OPC 小尺寸范围(300~500 nm)的颗粒数浓度也高,二者结合可以表明出现的纳米颗粒的尺寸都比较小。相反,CPC 颗粒数量浓度较低,OPC 在较大尺寸范围(>1000 nm)的颗粒数浓度也高则可能表明存在更大的颗粒和/或纳米颗粒发生团聚。这些纳米颗粒与大颗粒和/或纳米颗粒产生团聚体的假设可通过 TEM 和 SEM 进行验证。

2. 选择性

空气中的纳米颗粒存在于许多工作场所,它往往有多个来源,如燃烧、汽车尾气排放等。粒子计数器通常不能给出颗粒源或成分信息,很难区分偶然产生和加工产生的颗粒。CPC 和 OPC 可用来确定纳米材料来源,同时将滤膜上的样本用于纳米颗粒尺寸、形状、化学成分的验证从而区分偶然的纳米颗粒和加工过程中产生的纳米颗粒。

3. 局限性

根据颗粒排放来源的数量和种类不同,气溶胶数量浓度测量时常常会有数量级上的差异,连续不同季节监测多日可以更好地了解空气颗粒数量浓度背景值以及纳米材料加工过程颗粒物释放的变化。

CPC 的动态范围上限是 100000 P/cm^3,可以通过在入口处安装稀释器的方法使 CPC 测量范围扩大。

通过 TEM 和 SEM 分析及能谱分析可以提供纳米颗粒的形态以及元素构成信息,如相关方法 NIOSH 方法 7402 和 7404(NIOSH,1994 年)。然而,当膜上颗粒物太多时 TEM 和 SEM 分析可能受到影响,或者颗粒物浓度低也无法准确的评估颗粒物特征。

另外区域样品数据收集尽可能地靠近释放源,以便更加准确的测量纳米颗粒的释放及找到最有可能影响工人暴露的位置,这些结果可以作为存在暴露释放的证据,需要实施一定的控制措施。

欧盟第七框架计划(EU-FP7)纳米材料风险管理研究团队(Managing Risks of Nanomaterials,MARINA)推荐方案:

可分为三部分:工作场所信息收集,基础评价和深入评价。为了使收集的数据可有效用于后续的风险评估和流行病学研究,所有信息需要认真整理并存储在纳米暴露及其相关信息数据库(Nano Exposure and Contextual Information Database,NECID)。目前没有生产纳米材料或偶尔产生纳米颗粒等工作场所同样需要评估,该评估草案也适用于这些场所。

4. 工作场所相关信息收集

确定工作场所中确实有纳米颗粒释放,选择释放量大、潜在暴露可能性大的区域进行评估。这些信息可用于后续数据共享和比对、建立暴露模型、获得暴露阈值,还可确定研究重点。应调查和记录下述信息:

◇ 公司名称;
◇ 位置,地址,周围环境;
◇ 生产流程,如合成、处理、打包等;
◇ 使用的纳米材料,如化学成分、纯度、表面修饰等;
◇ 材料使用量;
◇ 物料安全数据表(MSDS);

◇ 任务评估；

◇ 处理材料的设备类型；

◇ 个人防护措施(Personal Protective Equipment,PPE)的使用；

◇ 通风,房间大小；

◇ 监测位置选择；

◇ 人造纳米材料的释放源辨识；

◇ 纳米颗粒的其他来源:柴油机,加热器,高温炉等；

◇ 工人数量；

◇ 暴露时间；

◇ 暴露频率。

5. 基础评价

获得空气中颗粒浓度和颗粒类型的初步定量评估。使用一个非纳米尺寸的选择性的实时便携式颗粒数量浓度检测仪器,如 CPC,仪器使用前及使用后要进行零点检查;使用滤膜或者一些专业设备收集电镜样品,如纳米尺寸气溶胶收集器,使用带有能谱的电子显微镜对收集的样品进行分析,确认纳米颗粒的存在;使用个体监测仪(如 MiniDISC,Nanotracer)监测个体暴露情况。

厂区背景值的测定应在生产前或生产后进行,或者在远离厂区的地方测定。具体根据仪器类型和生产过程(持续或间断)而定。监测时长应保证数值达到一个相对稳定的状态。这种状态比较难以达到,因为其他来源颗粒物的出现,背景浓度会出现波动。最好的方法是使用相同的仪器同时测定近厂区和远厂区的背景值。同时还应考虑其他来源的纳米颗粒,如具有致癌性的柴油机颗粒。还应考虑在某种状况下释放的背景气溶胶纳米颗粒清除的情况。

与背景值相比,如果检测到高浓度的纳米颗粒,则需使用新的暴露评估方法再次监测。如果纳米颗粒释放源自一些偶然事件,则需排除这个事件后重新评估。

监测时需要记录颗粒物数量浓度的均值和峰值。如果生产过程持续时间超过30 min 或 1 h,则监测时间应包含整个工作过程,同时要记录监测时间,保存原始数据记录。

依据电镜分析结果,评估纳米颗粒物的数量(无,少,多)以及团聚状态(原始,团聚,聚集,疏松),保存电镜图片。

基本评估设备：

◇ 个体监测仪:如 DISCmini；

◇ 近厂区监测仪:CPC 或扩散荷电装置,以及用于监测大颗粒的 OPC；

◇ 远厂区监测仪:CPC 或扩散荷电装置；

　　◇ 电镜样品收集：如静电除尘器。
文件资料：
　　◇ 监测位置；
　　◇ 背景监测位置；
　　◇ 温度和相对湿度；
　　◇ 仪器，包括硬件设备、流量、检测限等；
　　◇ 采样时间；
　　◇ 质量控制方法（如校准、零点监测等）；
　　◇ 记录所有的活动（工人工作，开、关门，车辆等）；
　　◇ 电镜样品收集的时间、地点、均匀性；
　　◇ 背景颗粒数量浓度（峰值和均值）；
　　◇ 监测位置颗粒数量浓度（峰值和均值）；
　　◇ 平均时间；
　　◇ 典型电镜图片；
　　◇ 电镜图片分析（是否有纳米颗粒、团聚、聚集或疏松）；
　　◇ 能谱对元素成分分析；
　　◇ 原始数据。

　　6. 危险信息评估

　　如果监测结果中显示有纳米颗粒，但其颗粒数量浓度与背景值相比并没有显著差异，则需要获得其危险性信息。如果不知道纳米颗粒的危险性信息或该纳米颗粒的危险性比背景颗粒大很多，则需要精确评估以确定纳米颗粒在目前浓度没有潜在危害。我们需要强调它与危险评估的联系，并把相关信息告知参与危险评估的项目组成员。

　　7. 深入评价

　　如果确定有纳米材料释放，则要深入收集各项信息，包括颗粒数、尺寸分布，表面积浓度以及质量浓度/质量尺寸分布。
　　包括如下仪器：
　　◇ 颗粒数尺寸分布：SMPS，FMPS，ELPI，NPS500；
　　◇ 单颗粒数量浓度：DISCmini；
　　◇ 近厂区和远厂区颗粒数浓度（平行监测）：CPC，扩散荷电装置（DISCmini，Nanotracer）；
　　◇ 质量浓度：TEOM；

◇ 质量尺寸分布：BLPI，DLPI，MOUDI，阶式碰撞采样器；

◇ 表面积浓度：NSAM，Aerotrack，LQ1。

需根据气溶胶的特征、最合适的度量以及现有监测方法的优点和局限性确定监测指标和使用仪器，仪器使用前、后应进行零点校准。最后的结果应给出质量浓度和表面积浓度的平均值及峰值。监测时间可以跨越整个工作时间，如果工作时间是一个持续的时间，则可以监测 30 min 或者 1 h。可通过查阅参考文献确定监测时间，保存原始数据。颗粒数尺寸分布数据可分为两类：≤100 nm 和＞100 nm。颗粒数量浓度监测应及时进行评价以防止到达暴露限值。推荐参考德国社会意外保险职业安全与健康研究所(IFA)使用的限值(IFA，2012 年)：

◇ 尺寸在 1～100 nm 的密度大于 6000 kg/m³ 的金属、金属氧化物和其他生物界存在的颗粒状纳米材料：数量浓度不超过 20000 个/cm³；

◇ 尺寸在 1～100 nm 的密度小于 6000 kg/m³ 的生物界存在的颗粒状纳米材料：颗粒数量浓度不超过 40000 个/cm³。

4.5　空气中人造纳米材料的暴露评价

如前所述，进行暴露评价有诸多原因。如果目的是针对生产场所的工人进行暴露评价，则需要确定一系列的具体监测指标：怎样从背景气溶胶中辨别人造纳米材料，我们应该监测的尺寸上限是多少，怎样监测纤维，怎样处理时空变化，应做多少次监测，每次监测多长时间，仪器的监测局限(如缺少个人监测仪)。

4.5.1　监测指标

常规的颗粒物暴露监测是进行个体质量测定，这也是一些现行标准的制定基础。然而，这种方法并不适用于纳米颗粒，因为纳米颗粒的质量远小于大颗粒[93]。超细颗粒物(dp＜300 nm)和纳米颗粒物的毒理学机制尚未清晰，所以不确定哪一项指标(如颗粒数量浓度、质量浓度、表面积、颗粒形貌或其他)最适于评价其潜在健康危害。已有研究表明同种化学成分的纳米颗粒比表面积的增加可使其生物活性增加[94]，因此，颗粒表面积和个数比质量更适用于评估纳米颗粒对健康的影响。

暴露监测、颗粒物检测以及评价需要考虑指标的稳定性。质量浓度不会因为颗粒的团聚或者团聚体密度的改变而发生变化，但是表面积和颗粒数量浓度会发生很大的变化。

监测可吸入纳米颗粒暴露的有效方法是检测气溶胶的个数、表面积和质量浓度。现有设备可以测定这些参数以及一些其他参数，但是这些设备不适宜监测个体暴露，需精确、便携和性价比高的设备才能够监测个体暴露[93]。对于肺部沉积表面积监测(基于扩散电荷,如 iDiSC)、颗粒个数尺寸分布监测和化学成分监测(基于配有 SEM-EDX 的热泳采样器)此类设备正在研发中。此外,单一参数并不适用于所有的纳米材料,理想的方法是选择与健康效应相关的参数。选定的参数应容易测量、灵敏度高,易与背景值区分,同时纳米颗粒的化学组成很重要。

目前有一些研究针对纳米材料职业暴露限值(OELs)的评价方法,是以质量浓度和目前存在的数量浓度为基础的方法。例如,根据国立职业安全与健康研究所(NIOSH) 5040 条例(美国 1994 年),其推荐的评估是根据大量航空碳浓度测量来做分析。美国环球航空公司(TWA)相关的每 8 小时 7 μg/m³ 碳浓度暴露水平是在量化上限(LOQ)分析方法的基础上建立的(NIOSH 5040)。NIOSH 认为此相对水平可能无法完全保护工人的健康但有助于使发展中国家肺部疾病的风险最小化。NIOSH 也公布了纳米级 TiO_2 的职业暴露限值是 0.3 mg/m³(NIOSH,2011 年)。

4.5.2 背景及其他来源的纳米颗粒

人类目前暴露于浓度范围从每立方厘米几百到几万的微粒环境中。这些颗粒来源于各种自然的和人为的因素,如森林火灾、交通、燃烧源等,在这些过程中产生的大小不同的颗粒同样也包括纳米颗粒。然而,它们的形态和化学成分一般会与人工纳米材料(ENM)有所不同。为了评估 ENM 暴露风险,我们需要区分不同来源的颗粒。

在特定职业环境中,需要确定纳米颗粒背景的来源(供热单位、铲车、吸尘器等),同时需要考虑室外的来源。欧洲化学品管理局(ECHA)认为可以用三种方法确定背景来源,例如(ECHA,2011 年):

(1) 在活动发生之前,用同样的仪器在事件/活动发生的同一地区采样。这种方法被称为"近场"的方法。这意味着,以不同时间点的事件和非事件的相关记录测量(即背景)来确定颗粒水平和事件之间的合理关系。

(2) 在预期仅有背景值的地区,用相同的仪器进行数据采样测量。这种方法被称为"远场"方法。这样的位置可以定位在室外或者在建筑物/实验室的远端一处位置。

(3) 收集物理气溶胶微粒样品做离线分析,可通过成分,形态或者 SEM/TEM 以及 EDX 分析方法提供依据,以确认观察到的峰浓度所对应的是确定的纳米材料释放事件。同时使用上述监测方法,通常能更成功地识别 ENM 释放和背景气溶胶之间的关系。

NIOSH 提出当背景浓度过高或波动较大时,从实际测量数据中扣除背景颗粒数浓度是比较困难的。建议通过同时设置滤膜过滤器收集释放材料,再使用透射电子显微镜(TEM)进行测量分析确定,可以给出颗粒大小的分布结果。TEM

可以联合能谱仪(EDS)进行元素组成的测定,以此来确定纳米材料释放的种类。

区分不同的来源颗粒最合适的方法,取决于测量目标,设备的可用性,实际情况(通风,其他来源等)和测量的时间等,当然也需要关注一下环境背景,例如是否应该从结果中减去或单独报告? 无论采用哪种方法,这都需要进行清晰地描述和记录。

4.5.3　需要考虑颗粒的大小上限

ENM 的大小上限,通常被认为是 100 nm(至少在同一个尺度上)。空气中 ENM 易于团聚,或者在高浓度($>10^6$颗粒$/cm^3$)时与背景颗粒结合互相结合在一起,即初级颗粒尺寸可能是低于 100 nm,而团聚物的大小可能会超过 100 nm。

欧盟委员会已经发布了关于纳米材料如何定义的提议[EC 2011]。根据该提议,"纳米材料"是指一种天然的,偶然产生的或人工制备的材料颗粒,处于游离状态,或呈结合的团聚状态存在形式,一维或更多维度尺寸在 1~100 nm 尺寸范围之间。

4.5.4　纤维状或高长径比的纳米材料

传统上石棉等这种具有特定的形状和组成纤维气溶胶暴露的评估,是通过测量空气中的纤维数量浓度进行评估(ECHA,2011 年)。此方法依赖于光学显微镜来人工纤维计数。

由于碳纳米管的直径很小,在光学显微镜下监测不到,只能在成束状聚集时才可能被检测到。因此需要用更高放大倍数的工具如 SEM 和/或 TEM 来观察,但实际上这样会增加计数时间。目前关于最合适的做法还没有达成共识,也没有给出具体的指导建议,但是,应该在评估中特别指出纤维成分可能存在的这些问题。

4.5.5　浓度随空间和时间变化

随着新粒子释放、形成、沉积、团聚、空气流动等变化,气溶胶颗粒的浓度和粒度分布也在不断改变。由于它们受到环境气溶胶颗粒的结合清除和/或彼此碰撞,从释放的位置到人体暴露的位置,ENM 的粒度分布和数量浓度都会发生很大变化。其中,影响颗粒大小分布变化及数目浓度变化的关键因素是颗粒释放时的浓度、换气速率以及背景颗粒浓度和尺寸大小。在气溶胶中 ENM 仍然以某种化学形式存在于环境中,它们看似是由背景颗粒扣除,实则是在空气中以形成大的颗粒形式分布于环境气溶胶中。

颗粒尺寸分布和颗粒数浓度随着时空发生变化,这对释放暴露监测提出了更大的挑战。同时表明,这需要不同水平的监测,包括静态和个体暴露,以及空气中的颗粒的化学组成分析等方面的信息。已经有数据表明,通常个体暴露水平监测会比静态位置测量的暴露水平更高(ECHA,2011 年)。因此,便携易用的便携式个人采样器的需求日益增加,而近年来这些测量设备已开发出来(Nanotracer,迷你盘)。在此期间,使用静态测量设备也是必要的选择。

在测量过程中,对影响测量的相关信息进行详细记录和阐释是非常重要的。即一般在测量期间整个过程中的情况,包括活动,是否使用了相关防护设备或措施,如通风情况,防护口罩情况等都需要记录。

第 5 章　纳米颗粒暴露防护建议

为了降低职业暴露风险,需要针对呼吸道及皮肤暴露情况进行必要的个人防护,同时从技术及组织管理层面制定严格的规章制度,消除或降低暴露风险发生的可能性。

5.1　控 制 方 法

5.1.1　概述

与宏观尺度的材料相比,纳米颗粒拥有独特的理化性质,使它们在工作场所的空气中也展现出与大颗粒的不同。然而从工程控制的角度来看,这种差异并不是最重要的。美国国家职业与卫生研究院认为,对于大多数流程和工作任务,与降低气溶胶暴露时使用的方法类似,控制纳米颗粒的空气接触可以用常规的工程控制技术来实现。

纳米颗粒暴露工程控制技术可以在现有的气溶胶暴露控制经验和基础上建立,目前气溶胶暴露控制技术已经应用于超细颗粒物暴露控制领域,比如焊接、炭黑或者病毒接触。我们可以对现有技术进行修改或重新设计以适用于纳米颗粒的暴露控制,如常规的通风设施,密闭设施,过滤设计等。

纳米颗粒的大小和质量对其随气流运动,沉积和聚集/团聚行为有一定的影响,与微米级颗粒物相比,纳米颗粒可随气流运动,甚至会湍流运动。颗粒物的弛豫时间是一种监测颗粒物遵循流速变化的方法,小于 100 nm 的颗粒比 1 μm 的颗粒小一至两个数量级。实际情况是,纳米颗粒很多时候在空气中的表现和大气颗粒物不一样,除了不会从表面反弹之外,更像大分子。纳米颗粒没有表现出重力沉降和表面沉积是因为布朗运动、湍流扩散、静态电场及热泳动。这种沉积和方向无关,颗粒物形成聚集体的过程导致随着时间延长颗粒数量浓度减小,但是并不改变质量浓度。在极高的浓度环境下(10^6 颗粒/cm^3 或者更高),从卫生学的角度分析,团聚可能会产生更大的影响。

国际纳米科技委员会(International Council on Nanotechnology,ICON)调查了世界各地纳米技术产业现状(2006 年),其中已报告的环境健康和安全措施,在处理化学物质方面与常规的安全措施没有明显的差异。大部分组织报道,在提高纳米环境健康和安全研究中最大的阻碍就是信息缺乏,因此,产业和政府针对环境健康的安全措施及指导工作十分重要。值得注意的是,关于"最佳措施"和纳米材料风险管理框架的指导条例是很少的,目前只能基于经验研究,即现有知识和专家经验。ICON 的研究只包括研究实验室和制造厂,并不包括诸如消费者和废物管理措施等环节。

5.1.2　风险控制方法

跟传统的暴露情况相似,大多数的纳米颗粒刚释放时会形成一个短暂的峰值。可以用观测和专业评价等定性评估方法来辨识释放源的具体位置。潜在释放源的释放频率和浓度可以用常规的气溶胶光度计进行检测。对于毒性可能较强的颗粒,可以选用灵敏度更高的仪器,比如凝聚核粒子计数器(CPC)。结合这些评估方法和研究步骤,比如利用影像记录同时进行的方法,可以为减少颗粒释放提供非常有价值的参考。

许多纳米颗粒商品以悬浊液形式出售,这是为了稳定材料,避免产生团聚并减少可能的释放暴露情况,而从干粉状态制成悬浊液过程中可能存在释放暴露,这也是需要考察的过程。

安全措施

实验室:使用凝结核粒子计数器应该可以确定控制是否有效。

生产场所:定性风险评估方法作为初步风险评估,包括外观检查,辅以合适的烟雾探测器,与操作人员讨论并评估可能的释放源及释放估计量。

在一些场所中,也可以通过观察灰尘积累量来找到颗粒释放源信息。对防护控制措施进行对应的评估也是工厂必要的工作内容。

5.1.3　纳米颗粒的过滤

各种传统设计的多孔过滤介质在过滤性能方面很相似,与过滤媒介特性和空气流量无关。对于足够大的颗粒(大于几微米),其渗透率接近零。随着颗粒尺寸的降低,渗透率增加,并在某一个尺寸表现出最大的渗透率,之后随着颗粒粒径的减小,渗透率逐渐降低,这种降低是由扩散沉积导致的。

传统纤维过滤介质最大能够渗透的纳米颗粒粒径约 300 nm,主要取决于空气流速和过滤纤维的直径大小,所以过滤器以该粒径尺寸的过滤效率进行分类,其他粒径的颗粒渗透率较低。最近发现对过滤介质进行预处理使之带上电荷,如对应普遍使用的面具和口罩,结果使 300 nm 颗粒渗透率降低,而粒径 30～70 nm 的颗粒则有了最大的渗透率。目前普遍认为,相对于颗粒的质量浓度暴露,数量浓度是一个更重要的健康风险评估参数,这可能导致以往对防护面具保护性能的过高估计,因为通常面罩是用 300 nm 大小的颗粒渗透数据进行评价。很有趣的是随着颗粒粒径变小,它们的行为越来越像分子,过滤效率也会接近于零。

颗粒尺寸产生的另一个影响是,小尺寸颗粒导致滤器的压降会比同样质量的大尺寸纳米颗粒增加得更快;与大的颗粒相比,滤膜上吸附亚微米级的颗粒会导致过滤器压降增大。

一般认为,过滤纳米颗粒不需要特殊开发新技术,已有的商业过滤介质可以成功应用于工业卫生环境。过滤性能可以用现有方法进行评估,例如标出适用的颗粒尺寸范围、控制措施等,并且也可以用现有理论进行模拟预测。对于预先处理的过滤介质,可能在基于标准检测方法的评级中高估了其过滤性能。

5.1.4　技术控制措施

一般将消除或降低工作场所中颗粒的释放作为技术控制的首要方向,包括密闭隔绝,加装局部排气设备,最好的方法是封闭颗粒的释放源,如果实现完全隔绝有困难,则可根据具体操作情况加装带有换气设备的洁净工作区,局部通风需要与总通风系统相配合,从而达到最好的净化效果,同时,通风系统的合理使用和维护是确保净化效能的必要条件。

对于清除进入通风系统中的纳米颗粒,需要使用过滤器,包括多级高效颗粒空气滤器(High Efficiency Particulate Air Filter,HEPA)及超低渗透空气过滤器(Ultra Low Penetration Air Filters,ULPA)。欧盟标准 EN 1822-1 至 EN 1822-5 提供了测定过滤效率的检测方法,即测定最易穿透粒径(Most Penetration Particle Size,MPPS)值为 120~250 nm 的颗粒的渗透率。通常将空气滤器分为有效滤器(Efficient Particulate Air Filter,EPA),高渗透和低渗透空气滤器。表 5.1 给出了滤器的分级数据。

表 5.1　根据欧盟标准及标准草案对高效滤器分级汇总

EN 1822-1:1998		滤器分级	prEN 1822-1:2008
渗透性			渗透性
整体值	局部值	过滤级别	整体值
15	—	E10	≤15
5	—	E11	≤5
0.5	—	E12	≤0.5
0.05	0.25	H13	≤0.05
0.005	0.025	H14	≤0.005
0.000 5	0.002 5	U15	≤0.000 5
0.000 05	0.000 25	U16	≤0.000 05
0.000 005	0.000 1	U17	≤0.000 005

注:整体值参见 EN 1822-5:2000 或 prEN 1822-5:2008 中的过程描述;
局部值(泄露)参见 EN 1822-4:2000 或 prEN 1822-4:2008 中的过程描述。

关于控制颗粒释放技术措施的相关研究较少,已有的研究显示,尽管通过使用设计合理、安装规范的工程控制措施可以保护工人不暴露于纳米颗粒,但十分有必要监测工厂空气中的颗粒物浓度,并对通风及过滤系统进行良好的维护,从而避免工作环境中存在渗漏或者滤膜过载导致的过滤失效情况。

1. 呼吸防护

呼吸过滤器材常用于过滤受污染空气中的颗粒成分。熔喷纤维、介电材料及玻璃纤维等都作为过滤膜广泛用于呼吸防护器材中。按照国际通用的 EN 标准评估呼吸防护的性能,EN 143 可用于评价滤膜或半面罩。性能通常分为三个等级,一级为低防护,二级为中等防护,三级是高防护,使用超过 1 μm 的多分散气溶胶作为渗透评测材料。

一些研究工作对防护装置进行了评价,如对 10～400 nm 的石墨烯纳米材料防护效果的评测显示,传统的玻纤和介电纤维对纳米材料的防护都十分有效。介电材料铝膜的半面罩防护效果评估显示,其对 40～400 nm 的多分散 NaCl 颗粒气溶胶过滤有效,使用单分散气溶胶颗粒监测时,发现 40 nm 的颗粒渗透效果最强。

对于工人而言,常规 N95 半面罩并不总是具有很好的过滤效果,对 30～70 nm 的颗粒具有最大的渗透性,这表示防护面罩对这部分颗粒防护欠佳。从理论模拟结果来看,机械过滤器对于尺寸在 300 nm 左右的颗粒具有最高峰值的渗透率,然而,像 N95 这种采用带电荷的滤膜的面罩,最高渗透峰值降低到纳米尺寸。对多种型号不同流量的呼吸过滤器的性能进行检测,结果显示直径为 20～100 nm 的颗粒渗透效果的变异系数为 0.10～0.54。一项研究结果显示,N95 呼吸过滤器在 85 L/min 的流量下,纳米颗粒有至少 5% 的渗透率,这一数值基本代表了工作场所呼吸过滤器的效率。尺寸小至 1 nm 的纳米颗粒通过玻璃纤维滤膜的过滤效率,可以用颗粒粒径凝聚核计数器(PSM-CNC)进行系统测量,可监测过滤中湿度及电荷对不同尺寸纳米颗粒的影响。结果显示,对于 100 nm 以下的纳米颗粒,过滤效率受到颗粒电荷的影响而与湿度无关;对于小于 2 nm 的颗粒,渗透性随着颗粒粒径降低而升高。此外,佩戴的舒适性,维护及佩戴者的使用次数等对暴露风险都有很大影响。许多国家都对不同等级、类型的呼吸器的影响因素进行标识,这些或多或少都与过滤效率有关。因此,从职业健康防护的角度,呼吸器的防护效果一般用呼吸防护因子来定义,而不只是取决于过滤效果,例如,佩戴时对脸部的贴合舒适性对人造纳米材料暴露防护效果有很大的影响,TSI 公司提供了用于检测贴合舒适度测试的仪器(TSI PortaCount® 与 N95-Companion™),通过在呼吸器内外位置处取样进行检测,这包含了滤膜本身渗透性也包含了因脸部贴合性导致的泄露情况,是检测呼吸器防护效果和最坏情况下的暴露数据。而对于半面罩来说,通常很明显的暴露风险就是来自于脸部和面罩之间的贴合程度因素。

2. 防护服

研究发现使用机织纤维与普通纤维介质作为滤膜的过滤效果类似,粒径为 $100\sim500$ nm 颗粒具有最大的渗透性,且随颗粒粒径减小而升高。并且聚乙烯无纺布(Non-woven Polyethylene Textile)对纳米材料的阻挡比棉和纸的效果更好。因此,应该避免使用棉类材料制作防护服。这些检测是使用正向气流进行的测试,与测定滤器过程相似。根据 $30\sim80$ nm 的石墨烯颗粒的研究结果,高密度聚乙烯纺织材料比棉与纸类材料防护效果更好。2008 年 11 月纳米材料安全生产和使用国际会议(NANOSAFE 2008)的研究结果显示,通过对石墨烯、TiO_2 和铂(Pt)等纳米材料进行不同防护装置的实验测试,发现非编织织物类材料气密性好,制成的防护服对 Pt、TiO_2 纳米材料的防护效果比棉和高分子聚丙烯类材料的防护效果更好。对于手套类产品,丁腈橡胶、氯丁橡胶制成的手套在持续数分钟的暴露下,对 10 nm 的 Pt、TiO_2 纳米材料防护效果更好。

3. 管理规范

纳米材料已经广泛应用于工业生产,已有的风险评估还远远不够,同时,还缺少明确的纳米材料风险评估规范。目前已有的相关研究主要集中在技术可行性上,很少有以风险控制为目标的指导规范。ICON 2007 年对已有的相关文献进行了综合比较,这些资料主要推荐使用针对细颗粒物气溶胶防护的规范文件,建议使暴露的可能性降到最低,而目前防护手套等过滤装置的有效性仍然存在很大的不确定性。

在缺少暴露阈值及暴露测量结果的情况下,通常在工作场所中利用分组控制(Control Banding)进行职业暴露评估,比如分成毒性风险组及暴露组,已经有这些领域的研究工作探讨。另一项关系到风险控制的内容是材料安全性数据表,该数据表对纳米材料的特性专门进行了探讨。

5.1.5　其他事项

1. 能见度

众所周知,不能仅凭视觉进行估计粉尘浓度。能见度取决于光照强度和车间结构,背景以及颗粒尺寸和浓度。如果可见,可吸入的颗粒仅仅看似为阴霾,而不是单个粒子。当其他因素不变时,随着粒子变小,其浓度需要升到非常高才能看到。据报道,氧化铝纳米颗粒在空气中浓度高达几克(每立方米)时,空气看起来仍然是透明的。因此在前期调查中暴露评估人员不能仅凭肉眼可见去判定是否有大量颗粒释放。因此,在任何暴露评估中,合适的粒子探测器是不可缺少的。

2. 表面沉积

当有扰动发生时,表面沉积的颗粒也可能成为空气中游离颗粒的二次来源。利用半经验模型,可以计算颗粒沉积垂直表面的速度。

5.2　针对碳纳米管(CNTs)的防护建议

5.2.1　工程控制

避免暴露于碳纳米管(CNT)或者碳纳米纤维(CNF)最有效的方法之一是在设计或者设定操作前期以及下游使用过程中减少暴露,将风险最小化(参考NIOSH 网站:www.cdc.gov/niosh/topics/PtD/)。这可以通过建立过程安全管理(Process Safety Management,PSM)完成。PSM 使项目或系统的发展得到了很好的运行和维护,确保在使用具有潜在危害的仪器设备时降低风险。PSM 项目的一个必要部分是在暴露于 CNT 或 CNF 前分析可能存在的风险,以便于更好地设计或设定设备,减小暴露的潜在可能性。与此同时,PSM 项目考虑的要素应与OSHA 安全管理标准相一致[29 CFR 1910.119]。

在 CNT 或者 CNF 不能被低风险或者无害材料取代的情况下,则所有的设备应满足降低工人暴露风险的操作规范。由于 CNT 或 CNF 工作场所安全性数据有限,尚不确定工作场所的所有工人是否都呼吸暴露于 CNT 和 CNF,也不能确定是否都位于 NIOSH 推荐的 REL 数值之下,即 $1~\mu g/m^3$(8 小时 TWA)。然而,暴露控制技术例如隔离释放源及配备高效微粒过滤器的局部排风系统(Local Exhaust Ventilation,LEV),都能够高效的清除空气中的纳米颗粒(包括 CNT 和CNF)。表 5.2 汇总了暴露控制系统的优、缺点。可根据纳米材料的数量、物理状态和工人接触材料的时间、频率选择合适的暴露控制系统(表 5.3)。例如,含有 CNT 或 CNF 固体的切割、打磨、钻孔过程应该使用局部排风等工程控制措施阻止气溶胶的释放,加工(如在反应容器中收集产品)和处理干燥的 CNT 或者CNF 应该密闭操作,并使用 HEPA 通风系统以更好地清除纳米颗粒,当材料使用量大、释放浓度高或重复工作时,应强制使用该系统。实验室处理 CNT 和CNF 应使用通风柜,例如低流量或者空气幕罩[36],或者使用手套箱来减少工人暴露。所有的暴露控制系统都应该进行优化设计,测试,并定期维护以保证最大防护效率。

表 5.2　暴露控制与隔离系统

分类	优点	缺点
A. 稀释性通风,无特定工程控制措施 　　在工作区域补充空气以稀释悬浮颗粒物。 　　适用于只有供热通风与空气调节需求的生产场所,不推荐控制 CNT 和 CNF 暴露	不需要局部排风或密闭设备; 在整个工作区域稀释或者分散空气中释放的颗粒物	没有从源头上控制暴露,空气释放可能蔓延整个区域,导致其他工人的暴露。 　　往往需要大量的气流来稀释污染物达到来降低职业接触限值,增加了操作成本。 　　当污染物的产生是合理范围并且材料毒性较低时才考虑使用
B. 局部通风系统(LEV) 　　在释放源加盖罩子来收集颗粒物,使工人呼吸区浓度显著降低。 　　包括: 　　B1 配备 HEPA 过滤系统的实验室通风柜(通常为 80～120 ft/min 的表面速度)。 　　B2 三级生物安全柜 　　B3 在释放源处使用能够操作手持工具的 LEV	通过在释放源处设计罩子来捕获释放气溶胶; 通常比稀释通风系统需要更少的整体通风率。 从工人呼吸区域排出气溶胶; 控制灵活,可用于多种任务或操作	LEV 要维持足够的空气量和吸除速度以确保颗粒物清楚效果; 工人必须经培训正确使用; 防护罩打开时需要调整到确保合适的罩面速度; 系统排气率需要严格评估确保合适的外排,同时做到最小的产品损失
C. 下游工作站 　　低速度(30 m/min)通风的下游小房间或密闭空间来容纳从工人呼吸区域排除的污染物	可手动操作	必须监测工作站的气量和控制速率并维持确保正确运行;工人技能操作或进行工作流程时会接触捕获的气溶胶;工人必须经培训正确使用
D. 封闭设计(隔离) 　　所有的过程或者工作任务是密闭的,减少工人暴露的机会 　　例如: 　　D1 手套箱隔离系统(配备 HEPA 过滤系统) 　　D2 三级生物安全柜	释放源隔离; 最小化外源污染; 需要工人使用 PPE 防护(例如口罩)	需要更多时间在封闭系统里移动材料和设备; 戴手套时很难操作材料; 限制了能够放在封闭箱内的材料尺寸; 需要定期清洗封闭系统

表 5.3　工程控制措施减少 CNT 和 CNF 的暴露

过程、活动	潜在暴露源和推荐的暴露密封度*
A. 实验及操作	暴露源:流化床、化学气相沉积等方法合成 CNT 和 CNF。包括:①合成后收集;②粉末转移;③清洗反应器;④从基底移走 CNT 和 CNF;⑤CNT 或 CNF 的纯化或者功能化(少量暴露)。 暴露控制:①实验室防护罩(配有 HEPA 过滤系统);②HEPA 过滤罩(手套箱)或者;③生物安全柜。打开反应器和收集时需要局部通风系统(LEV)
B. 实验室	暴露源:在超声 CNT 或者 CNF 悬浮液时,或者混合、称重、转移等操作少量的 CNT 或者 CNF 时。 暴露控制:①实验室防护罩(配有 HEPA 过滤系统);②HEPA 过滤罩(手套箱)或者;③生物安全柜
C. CNT 和 CNF 的操作和合成	暴露源:流化床,化学气相沉积等方法合成 CNT 和 CNF。包括:①合成后收集;②装袋;③粉末转移;④清洗反应器;⑤从基底移走 CNT 和 CNF;⑥CNT或 CNF 的纯化或者功能化(大量暴露)。 暴露控制:配备 HEPA 过滤器的专用通风系统,或/和配有 HEPA 过滤系统的 LEV。例如:称重站用通风袋,装袋操作使用下游工作站或者无通风空间,产品转移过程用透气袋
D. 生产和使用 CNT 和 CNF 功能材料和复合材料	1. 暴露源:混合、称重和转移少量的 CNT、CNF 的粉末或者分散液包括:①CNT 或者 CNF 连接到基底和包被;②在表面使用 CNT 或者 CNF。 暴露控制:①实验室防护罩(配有 HEPA 过滤系统);②HEPA 过滤罩(手套箱)或者;③生物安全柜。 2. 暴露源:操作大量的 CNT 或者 CNF 粉末,包括与基底的颠倒混合;还有旋转、扭曲、编织 CNT 成束、布等或对其喷洒进行表面包被等。 暴露控制:过程控制中的隔离技术如专用通风柜或者防护罩等,例如:称重站用通风袋,装袋操作使用下游工作站或者无通风空间,产品转移过程用透气袋。 3. 暴露源:打磨、钻孔,剪切或者其他用到含有 CNT 或者 CNF 复合材料的机械过程
D. 生产和使用 CNT 和 CNF 功能材料和复合材料	暴露控制:操作小片的 CNT 或者 CNF 功能材料:①实验室防护罩(配有 HEPA 过滤系统);②HEPA 过滤罩(手套箱)或者;③生物安全柜。 暴露控制:操作大量 CNT 或 CNF 功能复合材料,不适用防护罩,可使用:①配有 HEPA 过滤器的 LEV(可能包括 LEV 手持工具);②配有 HEPA 过滤器的下游工作站;③配有 HEPA 过滤器的防护罩或者;④湿式粉尘抑制技术,如湿锯加工

　　注:影响选择合适工程控制和其他暴露控制策略的因素包括材料的物理形式(干燥分散粉末、悬浮液)、工作时间、频率和使用 CNT 或者 CNF 的量等。必须测量空气中释放暴露量来确认控制的有效性。

5.2.2　工人教育与培训

建立 CNT 和 CNF 潜在暴露以及安全操作的工人教育和培训项目是防止产生暴露风险的关键。研究表明培训能够取得即时和长久的效果,其意义在于:①使工人能够了解到潜在危害信息;②使他们在学习知识和工作实践中,逐渐提高安全意识;③提供必要的技能来保证工人安全完成他们的工作;④建立条件保障和管理委员会等安全机构。这里建议按照 OSHA 危险废物操作和紧急处置标准方法(29 CFR 1910.1200)的要求培训和教育工人,并且按照文献[95]的建立指导条款。教育培训项目应该记录形成流程(例如标准操作流程 SOPs)用于:①控制方法达到暴露防护的要求;②向工人告知现场可能存在潜在的危害因素;③能够进行及时准确的评定 CNT 和 CNF 释放情况;④建立针对性的工程控制方法,并能准确实施;⑤建立危险控制管理的行为档案;⑥定期检查、维护防护措施。应该对流程管理进行周期性检查,随时更新,并且及时改善工人工作防护状况并落实到位。
教育项目也应该包括理论讲解及实际操作训练,如下:

◇ 潜在暴露于 CNT 或者 CNF 的健康风险;

◇ 安全操作 CNT,CNF 以及含有 CNT 和 CNF 的材料,最小化暴露损伤和皮肤接触,包括佩戴使用工程控制的口罩,手套等(PPE)以及良好的工作流程操作。

5.2.3　清洗和处理

在清洗 CNT、CNF 以及含有 CNT 或者 CNF 的表面时,应该制定保护工人避免暴露的详细流程。呼吸吸入和皮肤接触可能带来更大的风险,因为在清洗时可能会使 CNT 和 CNF 变成气溶胶(粉末形式)引起暴露,此时会比溶液中的 CNT 和 CNF 表现出更高的毒性,并且比包被的 CNT 和 CNF 材料毒性更高。

使用已知的暴露风险数据以及进行严格的操作流程,是处理表面污染的良好方式。防护清洁粉末性物质泄漏的标准方法同样适用于清洁碳纳米管或纳米材料的表面污染。这些措施包括使用 HEPA 过滤器、防尘布处理 CNT 和 CNF(粉末状)或者在处理之前润湿。含 CNT 或纳米液体的泄漏通常可以采用吸附材料或清洗盛放液体的器具。若采用真空清洗,应注意高效过滤器的正确安装并根据厂家说明使用合适的过滤器。此外,还应建立适当的废物处理(包括所有的清洗材料和其他如手套等污染的材料)规则并严格遵守。

5.2.4　个人防护服

目前还没有关于 CNT 和 CNF 暴露防护服或其他服装的统一标准,当可能有潜在危害时,劳动卫生管理部门或厂家应该为员工提供手部防护措施[OSHA

1910.138(a)]。目前,评估 CNT 和 CNF 皮肤暴露的数据十分有限,已有研究明确指出呼吸道和皮肤暴露于 SWCNT 具有潜在的危害,因此在操作和处理期间,工人应该在橡胶手套外层佩戴一层棉手套[25]。个人佩戴手套暴露 SWCNT 的量为 217~6020 μg 时,大多数 SWCNT 直接接触手套表面。对于不同类型纳米颗粒的实验研究发现,一定条件下的暴露可能导致皮肤渗透[96,97],并且颗粒的尺寸、形状、水溶性、表面包被等因素直接影响纳米颗粒潜在的皮肤渗透性[97,98]。体外研究表明,使用原代或者培养的人类皮肤细胞或者人工组织模型,SWCNT 和 MWCNT 能够进入细胞,引起前炎症因子的释放,诱导自由基产生引起氧化应激,并且导致细胞活力降低[3,99,100]。MWCNT 的表面性质决定其与细胞间的相互作用方式。当 CNT 团聚降低时,对于角质细胞的毒性增加[101]。对 SKH-1 小鼠进行局部给药(160 μg)发现,SWCNT 可引起局部炎症或者毛囊炎症,而在最低剂量时(40 μg)没有明显变化[102]。由此得出的结论是,未纯化的 SWCNT 的局部暴露剂量>80 μg/鼠能够诱发自由基、氧化应激以及炎症的产生。然而,同一种类型的 MWCNT 的皮肤毒性试验结果(Baytubes®)没有发现急性皮肤刺激或过敏反应,在根据 OECD 标准进行兔子测试时,发现只有轻微的眼刺激现象[103]。由于皮肤暴露 CNT 和 CNF 的数据比较有限,在以下情况最好穿着防护服和手套:各种清除或者控制 CNT、CNF 释放的技术措施效果都欠佳时,或有突发事件情况下。

如果穿戴防护服或者手套,要特别注意防护 CNT 和 CNF 接触受到磨损或者损伤的皮肤。基于已有的实验数据,在保护工人免受纳米颗粒暴露时透气面料制成的非织造织物可能比棉花或涤纶等织物更为有效[104,105]。纳米及亚微米颗粒穿透各种非编织物的研究结果发现,小于 100 nm 的氧化铁对医院实验服、防护服以及消防服等的透过比例很小,低于 5%[106]。在选择最合适的防护和舒适服装之间存在的矛盾——最高程度的防护服装(例如 A 级防渗透服装),同时也是长时间穿着最不舒服的;然而防护比较差的服装,却是穿戴最舒服的。商用手套对于皮肤暴露纳米材料的防护效果,依赖于手套的材质、厚度以及佩戴时的使用方式等(暴露时间或者其他化学暴露)[104,105,107]。同时,也需要考虑手套的耐久性,如暴露于分散成液体形式的纳米材料以及化学品等可能会降低使用寿命。当工人需要额外的防护时,可以采用双层手套(如丁橡胶腈、氯丁橡胶、乳胶等手套)加以防护。特别注意,也应该考虑采用适当方法脱去并处理污染的手套,以防止皮肤污染,手套也应该定期检查并且及时更换。

5.2.5　口罩

如果工程控制措施和工作时间不能将工人暴露的 CNT 和 CNF 减少到职业接触限值以下,那么工人应该佩戴口罩防护。在一定的工作情况下,特别是高浓度暴露(例如清理或者维护 CNT 和 CNF 设备、清理捕获 CNT 和 CNF 气溶胶的过滤系统)时,建议佩戴口罩。OSHA 的呼吸保护标准(29 CFR 1910.134)提供了自愿使用和必须使用口罩两种情况。当口罩用于工人防护时,OSHA 呼吸防护标准要求建立一个独立的呼吸保护项目,需包括:①佩戴口罩时工人工作执行能力的医学评估;②正规的人员培训;③定期检测工作场所暴露情况;④选择口罩的程序;⑤口罩测试;⑥口罩的维护,检查,清洗以及储存。应该定期评价该方案的有效性,口罩项目负责人应该是熟悉工作场所并懂得口罩各种缺陷的专业人员。

　　根据已发表的工作场所 CNT 和 CNF 监测数据,当对工人、工作场所和工程控制措施进行测试的时候,应该提供 NIOSH 许可的、带有过滤器的口罩或者配有95 或者 100 系列滤器的半面罩[108]。在浓度高于职业接触限值 10 倍的情况下,应提供一种测试良好的半面罩或者带过滤器的口罩进行防护。同时还应提供其他更高级别防护的口罩(见表 5.1)。

　　在选择口罩的时候,应该考虑工人可能暴露的颗粒尺寸大小[109],以及其他工作场所是否也存在气溶胶。基于这些信息,管理者可以决定选择一个具有较高指定防护指数(Assigned Protection Factor,APF)的口罩或选择一个具有较高过滤性能的口罩(例如,从 N95 改为 P100)。对 N95 过滤式呼吸防护口罩过滤性能的研究发现,40 nm 左右颗粒的平均穿透率在 1.4%～5.2%之间,表明 95 和更高效过滤口罩可有效捕获 CNT 和 CNF[47,110]。最近的研究也表明,正如单纤维理论预测的那样,使用 NIOSH 认可的过滤式呼吸防护口罩可以有效地捕获小于 20 nm 的颗粒[47,111]。

第6章　职业暴露风险评价方法

6.1　职业暴露因素和风险管理措施

纳米材料的暴露释放取决于物质和产物的特性、过程、工作活动条件和采取的风险管理措施。为了能够进行适当的工人暴露评估,需要获得如下与暴露源和暴露决定因素相关的信息:

- 这些物质用在哪里?(包括过程、活动及产物的描述);
- 混合物(制备)和物品的成分(包括大概的百分含量);
- 在物质中可能含有的有毒杂质;
- 物质怎样使用?(包括对工作活动导致的暴露以及使用数量的描述);
- 加工材料和最终产物中大概的百分含量;
- 暴露性质,即操作条件(包括工作类型、大致频率和持续时间,暴露的持续时间和频率);
- 在工作中,用到了哪些技术上的或者个人的风险管理措施,包括各种优化流程及良好维护的防护设备;
- 为了确保暴露防护措施得到实施而提出的相关管理建议(例如,缩短暴露时间、正确使用个人防护设备等)。

对于初步评估步骤,以上信息的详细程度可以相应降低,这应该与具体评估要求相关。对于更进一步的评估,则需要许多另外的细节用于后续暴露评价。

相关的纳米颗粒产品可以运用风险管理措施,例如通过把粉末转换成油脂包覆的粉末来减少漂浮粉尘的尘污,这可以通过生产者具体操作执行。风险管理措施可分层级进行,即STOP原则、代替(Substitution)、技术测定(Technical measures)、组织措施(Organisational measures)和/或个人措施(Personal measures)。

6.2　用测量和模拟的方法进行暴露评价

6.2.1　概述

人类职业暴露评价应该基于以下核心原则:

暴露评价应该以合理的科学方法为基础,对所做出的结论和假设的基础都应该给予合理解释,任何讨论过程都应以公开透明的方式呈现。

　　暴露评价应该描述在操作条件下特定活动过程中的暴露,以及与暴露场景相关的风险管理措施(Risk Management Measures,RMMs),包括相关的地点,特定人群。应该特别关注受到显著暴露的人群或者暴露现场。在可能的情况下,应该依据合理的,且是最高暴露情况下的典型现场状况进行暴露评价,能达到这种暴露水平的概率很小。为了找到合理的最高释放暴露情况,研究人员建议在一定的监测情况下,选用所获得的全部暴露数据中分布处于百分之九十的数值量。合理的最高暴露情况不应该包括极端使用或滥用造成的极高暴露情况,但是可以包括正常使用的上限,因为人们通常认为暴露控制没有效果或效果很差。人为事故、故障或者恶意滥用的极端暴露情况不应该作为正常暴露情况对待。定期的清洁和维护属于正常的使用范围内。

　　暴露评价应该通过收集必要的信息(包括从模拟的场景或者是模型中得到的)和评价信息(在质量和可靠性方面等等)来建立,这样能够得到可靠的暴露评价结论,且评估过程需要考虑不确定性估计因子。

　　在评估暴露风险管理措施有效性的过程中,应该考虑现场已有的暴露控制措施,对一部分暴露方案适用的风险管理措施可能不适用于其他的暴露方案。

　　暴露通常理解为外部暴露,定义为物质摄入总量,皮肤接触总量(以单位mg/cm^2表示暴露评价结果),或/和吸入量或者空气中的物质浓度。暴露应分为长期暴露和短期暴露,并比较各自的推算无效应阈值(Derived No Effect Levels,DNELs)。对于不同的评价,必须要测定其风险特征比率(Risk Characterisation Ratio,RCR),相当于获得暴露等级与 DNEL。

　　总的 RCR 值等于各 RCR 之和(＝呼吸 RCR＋皮肤 RCR)

　　指示性职业暴露限值(Indicative Occupational Exposure Limit,IOEL)时,某些条件下可用 IOEL 代替 DNEL。

　　暴露可以是单个事件、一系列重复事件或者连续暴露事件。评价时应该考虑到暴露的持续时间和频率、暴露途径、工人的习惯和工作活动以及技术过程。一个方案中工人有可能暴露于来自不同产物的物质,这可以理解为在工作场所中与来自不同暴露源的联合暴露有关。另外,在暴露评价和风险表征过程中,消费者的兴趣爱好应该在反映暴露情况的方案中进行评价阐释。

　　在暴露评估中,依次按照如下先后顺序进行暴露等级评价:
- 测量数据,包括对关键暴露决定因素的定量;
- 合适的模拟数据,包括对关键暴露决定因素的定量;
- 模型评估。

　　当然,这些优先顺序排列只是为了反映测量数据是否有代表性并且是否合理。在很多情况下,结合测量数据和建模方法能够进行恰当的评估,不确定分析可以帮助说明对暴露风险评价有最大影响的关键因素。

6.2.2　工作场所暴露评价的分级标准

有效的工作场所暴露数据在暴露评价过程中起着关键的作用,信息来源包括证明文件和由厂商及下游用户收集的、用于完成化学试剂指示条款的工作场所测量值(98/24/EC)。这样的数据,如果质量好并且有充足的信息支持,可适用于任何暴露典型方案,能比任何模拟都更好地反映真实的条件。在暴露评价的过程中使用这些暴露测量值,应该考虑许多因素(IPCS,2008 年):

- 这些数据与正在研究的场景对应吗?
- 这些数据有足够的相关信息支持,使得它们与方案的关联性可以比较吗?
- 数据是基于合适的样品和分析技术确保其监测灵敏性吗?
- 有足够多的有效数据值并且对评价的暴露方案是否有代表性?

有大量关于建立和实施暴露检测策略的指导,用以有效的评价风险管理措施,以及报道相关信息(OECD,2003 年)。通常建立暴露方案的过程不需要一开始就进行暴露监测,更确切地说,这个过程需要足够的有效暴露数据开展后续评价工作。如果完全没有数据,可以对源自模拟和模型的数据进行专业的判定。

为了评估暴露数据和信息的有效性和适用性,本指南总结了合理测定最高释放情况和典型暴露数值,目标是增强这些数据的可靠性。如果暴露评价的基础很弱,建议将这些表格增加更多的信息,而大多数建立暴露方案所需的有关信息种类都在表格中显示(见附录)。

6.2.3　需要的核心信息

在初级监测暴露方案中需要掌握以下关键因素:

- 物质的物理状态;
- 使用物质的物理状态;
- 蒸汽压(液体);
- 不同含尘度等级(固体);
- 合成的物质浓度;
- 封闭水平;
- 局部通风效率(LEV);
- 活动持续时间;
- 对这种物质需要信息:包括相关的参数、施加于该物质或者产品的能量,如果使用的量很小,则需要原料与空气接触的表面积参数。

对于潜在暴露评价,即使可能会用到个人防护设备,但一般不作考虑。但是当没有个人防护设备不能正常工作例外,例如处理腐蚀性物质的时候必须使用手套,或者接触石棉时一定要使用防尘口罩,否则会造成严重的健康风险。使用个人防护设备减少暴露是后续评价的工作内容。

6.2.4　测量数据的使用

我们要意识到有效的工作场所暴露数据不仅在建立暴露场景的过程中很重要,而且对于评价安全管理措施的有效性也很重要。因为暴露场景提供了足够的风险管理措施和操作条件,使得工作场所的暴露控制在物质 DNEL 以下。工作场所暴露监测是帮助管理人员确定从上游供应链获得的暴露控制建议的完整性和有效性。目前已经建立大量有关怎样建立暴露监测策略和执行评价推荐的风险管理建议的有效性指导(CEN 1995)。通常建立任何暴露场景的过程不需要一开始就进行暴露监测,更确切地说,这个过程需要重视从实际、模拟和模型得到的有效暴露数据。

在化学药品安全评价中,暴露评价的目的是在暴露现场获得与所描述的操作条件和风险管理措施有关的暴露等级。因为即使定义明确,暴露现场都会有很大的变化性,所以评价所谓的"合理的最糟糕的情况"暴露等级很重要。在暴露现场中最高等级暴露发生在特殊的情况下,可以导致比平均值更高的暴露,例如,在有限的自然通风下,高负荷生产率、高温条件等。这种合理的最高暴露情况发生概率很小,但实际上,它排除了明显在通常暴露之外的情况,例如严重事故后的暴露或工人不遵守指示的情况下的暴露,或不使用必需的风险管理措施的暴露。使用合理的最高的暴露值而不是最大或最坏情况的暴露值,可以减少暴露分布的偶然异常值的影响。

理想的情况应该是在明确的暴露现场有足够有效的暴露测量值,判断所选的风险管理措施和操作条件是否可以将暴露水平控制在 DNEL 以下。然而,这种判断的前提是:①任何暴露现场有足够且具代表性的有效数据;②数据质量较高,不能因为它们固有的不确定性就不使用。在这一方面,没有定义足够数据量有"多少"组成。建立暴露现场"有效的暴露测量值"是硬性规定,但可以假设暴露现场反映广泛的、一般的活动,可能不只是需要与特殊情况有关的暴露现场。

虽然测得的数据对于常用的物质有效,特别是那些被认为是危险的物质,但对于不常接触到的化学药品不一定适用。然而,对类似的物质和/或对暴露建模估算的合适测量数据可能是有效的。在很多情况下,暴露数据的不同形式都是有效的,但必须以一种涉及它们固有性质并按优先顺序排列的形式,把它们结合起来。

因为对测量数据作出判断的人可能是厂商或者进口商的代表、配方设计师、特殊组织的一个部门或者一个公司,在下文中统一称为评审员。在很多情况下,有一些必须测量的数据,这些数据可用以下方式得到:

• 测量数据的数据库,例如来自注册人在制造过程中的测量数据,或者政府、研究所拥有的数据库,如从验证检验得到的数据等。

- 在公共领域对职业暴露的调查(例如对一种物质、一个种类进行的调查);
- 在公共领域外,由制造商/进口商/供应商/贸易协会收集的关于一种物质的数据。

测量数据可能与物质本身或者类似的物质有关,这是最好的情况。或者,测量数据可以准确地呈现暴露现场的情况或者类似的情况(例如用胶合代替毛刷涂装)。对于暴露评估的目的,类似数据是基于相同操作的数据,如果没有类似的物质,就使用同一物质或者基于同样操作获得数据。一般认为大多数物质都有类似标志物,例如关于评价物质的数据不可用或者不充足,可以使用那些类似物的信息。有时候,根据优先数据排列中,有关标志物的数据可能没有同等的可靠性,但是可以提供比从模拟评估更有价值的信息。

当使用从类似物得到的数据时,厂商或者进口商必须确定这种估计能给出安全可靠的结果。例如,基于从较易挥发物得到的数据进行挥发性稍低物质的评估是安全可靠的,而基于从不易挥发物得到的数据去估计高挥发物质则不是安全可靠的,这导致了对风险的低估。譬如,假设在印刷行业中对用作洗涤剂的二甲苯的暴露评价是必需的,并且没有(或很少)测量数据可用,而如果描述同样活动或者另一种溶剂(有相同的物理化学性质,有稍高的挥发性,例如甲苯)的数据可用,那么这些数据就可以认为是类似的且可以实际使用的,但是基于二甲苯暴露的甲苯暴露评估是不可行的,因为甲苯无疑是更容易挥发的。挥发性在呼吸暴露中是一个非常重要的参数,应该调整其可比性。同样地,对于物质外排,例如氧化锌粉末,需要做出暴露评价,但是没有数据得到认同,那么用另外的以同样的方式处理的固体粉末的数据是可以接受的。这种情况下,应该考虑含尘量的可比性,如果没有含尘量的信息,就要考虑用颗粒尺寸代替含尘量。

高质量的、明确的关于使用物质过程的信息是解释测量数据,或者所得到模型数据的必要条件。通过各种途径充分表征暴露,得到暴露的最合理评价。为了这个目的,应该首先定义那些所需的决定性因素的核心信息。不管是否存在有用的辅助性测量数据,这些核心信息都应该考虑在任何暴露评估中。评审员需要仔细考虑相关的有效信息,即使测量数据不可用,为了使用暴露模拟,评审员仍需要所有的描述性数据。

6.2.5　测量数据的选择和分析

测量数据对于暴露现场应该具有代表性。建议首先检查从不同来源得到的数据是否可用,包括各种特定项目信息,同时参考已有的在该物质使用规范下进行的风险评价工作及相关科学文献所能提供的有用信息。收集不同的暴露数据,包括需要遵守国家健康和安全法律条款。因为数据收集目的可能会影响在研究暴露评价中的应用,所以其适用性需要得到评估。生产固体颗粒的尺寸和实际应用的含尘量相关性不大,所以使用与颗粒尺寸相当的物质得到数据,比用与含尘量相当的物质得到的数据会导致更大的不确定性。

当使用来自宽阔场所的暴露现场数据时,应该考虑这些数据是否具有代表性,是否可以用于暴露评价。对于化学产品的制造工序,不同工种之间有区别,例如一般的操作、装卸活动和维护工作之间是有差异的。

当可实施暴露测量时,应该尽可能把它们与在暴露现场中描述的操作条件和风险管理措施联系起来。这些信息包括:

• 反映个人暴露的原始数据(由单个数据点组成)列表:测量浓度、浓度单位、采样持续时间、暴露持续时间和频率、采样说明、在监测期间采用的分析方法和任务。

• 如有必要,用注解说明异常现象,数据应该包括个人的劳动班次、短期暴露或急性危害,或在引起显著暴露的条件下进行主要工作的最大暴露值。如果有充分的信息证明,定点采集的数据可以反映个人暴露,或者它们能提示个人暴露的保守估计信息,则这些定点采集数据可用于暴露评估,也就是说,在这种条件下的个人暴露水平应该比来自定点采样的低。

依据已有官方认可公布的标准进行收集和分析的数据,应具有质量保证措施,如 ISO/IEC17025:2005,清楚地描述了质量保证措施的要求、数据收集、方案的质量、实验室间质量保证、采样策略等。

用于验证数据可靠性和代表性的细节必须进行评估。注意事项如下:

◇ 采样的目的和时间?

◇ 数据是否包括了暴露现场中指定的过程、活动和风险管理措施?

◇ 测量的时候是什么样的条件? 例如正常的或者异常的。

◇ 数据是否按照有关化学试剂职业暴露的一般测量要求[例如 482:2006(CEN2006)]、测量策略[例如 EN689(CEN1995)]和有效的分析方法进行收集?

◇ 数据反映的是行业过去还是现在的活动情况?

◇ 数据反映一个公司的状况还是代表整个行业?

通常,为了充分描述一个工厂里单个工作活动的释放暴露,需要呈现采集至少6 个数据点,但是对于在一个行业的或一个部门里进行的工作活动,则需要考虑更多数据点(通常不少于 12 个)。风险评价所需的确切数据点个数在很大程度上取决于数据的可靠性,特别是需要在下述因素间进行平衡选定:数据的代表性,在数据集和待评价的情况下认为合适的水平,以及 DNELs(或者 DMELs)要求和测量暴露水平等级要求(见表 6.1)。暴露评价质量取决于基于离散的测量数据集的样本大小、数据的分散程度和数据集的均一性等,这与暴露场景现场的变化性有关。相关暴露估计值的可信程度随着样本数的增大以及分布变窄而增大。测量情景的广度现场的范围和它们与需要评估的情景现场是否配合匹配也很重要。对面积大的广阔场地的现场进行暴露评估需要更多的数据保证充分地包含了广阔的场景现场以及对潜在的有关子集的评估。另一个重要的因素是替代品样品的暴露水平和有关的暴露限值(合适的 DNEL)之间的比值,叫做 RCR。应该注意的是,一个公司的数据不可能代表整个行业部门。

表 6.1 给出了关于提高评估可靠性所需的采样点数量的经验法则,暴露数据和得到的风险特性比率(RCR)的变化和不确定性决定着所需采样点数量,因此应确保 RCR 小于 1。

表 6.1　为了确保真实的 RCR 值小于 1 所需的测量数

		0.5<RCR<1	0.1<RCR<0.5	RCR<0.1
		N	N	N
数据的变化性和不确定性	低∧	~20~30	12~20	6~12
	中+	~30~50	~20~30	12~20
	高*	>50	~30~50	~20~30

注:N 为样本数;

RCR 为风险特性比率;

数据的变化性和不确定性一方面与暴露中的真实变化有关(如测量变化表示),另一方面与相关数据是否能真实代表待评价情景有关。

* 高:一个高测量数据的几何标准差(GSD,例如>3.5)或者数据的典型性是否很好地代表评价现场状况,存在很大的不确定性。

+ 中:一个中等的测量数据几何标准差(例如 2~3.5)或者数据的典型性是有待考量的。

∧ 低:一个低的测量数据集的几何标准差(例如<2),该数据能很好地代表待评价现场。

可用以下例子进行说明,如果预期暴露中变化较高和/或与数据集典型相关的不确定性高,并且基于估计的合理的最高暴露值的 RCR 接近 1,则需要较多的数据点(例如>50)证明真正的 RCR 低于 1。但是,如果数据集与暴露现场符合度很好,暴露的变化有限并且与估计的最差情况比值 RCR 在 0.5~1 之间,数据集中12~20 个数据点就足以充分证明真正的 RCR<1。

为了得到呼吸暴露估计的典型结果,需要认真选择监测持续时间,另外,数据应该能够恰当地代表在整个过程加权平均基准期(一般 8 h)的暴露。

理想情况下,为了使数据能够作为暴露现场的典型,应该通过随机取样的方法进行数据采集。用非随机方法收集的数据对于暴露评价的结果来说是有偏移的,如使用最高暴露情况的取样作为合理计划的一部分。然而,这样的数据对于描述某些暴露现场是有用的,如果有足够的相关信息可用,它就可以用于后续分析。

数据总有偏差,但应该至少在定性方面确认数据内的显著偏差,并且进行相应处理。单独的偏差不应该从数据中删除,例如由于泄漏、溢出等原因的高暴露浓度的情况,应该认同这些偏差。

1. 颗粒尺寸

如果暴露在有粉尘的地方发生暴露的地方,应该提供有关颗粒尺寸分布的数据,颗粒在气管或肺泡中的不同分布决定了其生物摄取及这些颗粒的最终机体分布,反过来,机体沉积位置取决于颗粒尺寸大小的分布。可吸入粉尘(≤100 μm 或更小)、可吸入颗粒(≤10 μm 或更小)和超细或纳米颗粒(≤100 nm,即 0.1 μm)的百分数与健康有很大关系。对于有关粉尘的数据,应该提供取样采样方法所能获得的最小尺寸分布。

2. 皮肤暴露数据

影响到其他暴露方式的因素同样也影响潜在的皮肤暴露,如工作方式、环境条件和一些人为因素。污染物很少会均匀地分布在身体上,它可能只沾在保护皮肤的个人防护设备或者衣服上,或有可能存在于暴露的皮肤上,甚至是在保护服装下面的皮肤都可能受到污染。掌握污染物在身体上的分布有助于有效的风险评价,理想情况下,真正典型的暴露数据应该用于评价由皮肤暴露引起的健康风险。当暴露现场的测量数据可用的时候就使用这些数据进行皮肤暴露评价,不可用时,就用合适的模拟方法。

皮肤暴露数据应该包括以下信息:皮肤暴露的表面积(cm^2)、污染物的质量(mg)、单位面积的质量(mg/cm^2)、采样或暴露持续时间(min)、暴露频率(单个暴露情况在每天的发生次数)、采样方法和混合物的组分。要特别注意待评价物质的浓度,此信息应在描述暴露发生过程时进行补充。

辅助性的信息应包括所穿着的工作服的细节,一般工作服与防护服、装备的区别,以及个人卫生细节。由一般的不洁工作服引起的潜在暴露风险(实际上代表从前暴露现场的暴露),不应该影响当前暴露现场的结果。

关于皮肤暴露的测量数据不多,国际上"皮肤风险"(RISKOFDERM)项目是一个很好的参考资料,它产出大量的测量数据、报告和发表的文章,同时这个项目促进了潜在皮肤暴露评估专业模型的发展。

在处理腐蚀性或高热物质的过程中,必须使用防护手套和其他设备,如面罩、围裙等,同时需要良好的操作方法,以避免污染物与皮肤直接接触。因此,皮肤每天重复大量暴露的可能性不大。对于腐蚀性物质,在暴露现场中的重点是风险管理措施,而不是皮肤暴露风险评估。然而,可能需要对该物质的其他特性引起的影响进行评估。如果在使用腐蚀性物质的过程中,有制备稀释液/混合液的操作,这会导致皮肤产生暴露的风险,那么应该评估此物质的皮肤暴露,即不能忽视皮肤暴露问题。

对于易挥发物质,因为物质在皮肤上停留的时间短暂,皮肤暴露会减少。蒸发时间应与吸收率有关,可以给出吸收或从皮肤蒸发的外部污染物的相对百分比。如果工人与物质进行连续的直接接触,那么由于蒸发导致的暴露减少就不需考虑。另外,为了把物质的快速蒸发考虑在内,非保护下的皮肤暴露在暴露现场中应占主要部分。但是,物质从皮肤上无阻碍蒸发的场景也是有可能发生的,例如化工产业中的生产和进一步处理时。

3. 生物监测

生物监测数据可以用在暴露评估中,它可以提供总暴露(通过所有暴露途径)的性质和程度信息,使暴露评价信息更加丰富。生物监测资料作为一个额外的数据库,有助于更好地表征暴露,并进一步表明工作场所周围的控制措施和个人防护设备的有效性。然而,生物监测信息需要由经验丰富的从业人员认真分析,同时必须全面的提供相关信息,包括现场情况及相关步骤和任务。通过生物监测得到的被监测物质的半衰期,可以确定测量结果表示的是一天的暴露还是更长时间的暴露。例如,在某些情况下可以在一天结束时采一份血样,而在其他情况下,应该保留一整天的尿液样本(24 h)。

生物监测信息能反映实际暴露情况,即表示发生了暴露,并且已经被吸收到体内。然而,综合进一步获得的信息,比如采样地点和采样时间,可以提示暴露的主要途径或其他暴露途径占总剂量的相对比例。

生物监测信息应被视为等同于其他形式的暴露数据,例如空气污染物检测量。生物监测数据也必须达到一定的质量要求,即高质量的描述暴露情况且具有典型性。对于一些化合物,其生物监测方面已经得以很好的完善和描述(在方法学、分析数据的质量保证、控制参数和药代动力学方面)。然而,对于大多数物质,相关方法仍处于待完善阶段,如质量控制标准和测量程序缺乏。

还应该注意的是,生物监测结果反映个人对于该物质的总暴露,可能来自于任何相关途径,任何来源,即从消费产品和/或环境,而不只是职业暴露。尽管在许多情况下,职业暴露是最重要的,但是在混杂变量的情况下可能难以把生物监测数据和特定暴露情景联系起来。

暴露评价时生物监测数据应该提供相关参数,包括测量的确切参数,采样策略,例如在工作日结束时采样或是 24 h 采样,所测量物质的生物半衰期,对数据的解释及其他可能会有帮助的任何信息。生物监测数据作为吸入或皮肤暴露的数据应呈现相同的核心信息,使之与工作条件相关的结果得到正确解读。在有条件的情况下,应在生物监测水平和吸入(或皮肤)暴露水平之间建立联系,清晰呈现与呼吸和皮肤暴露水平、暴露持续时间和可能的健康影响相关的生物监测数据的含义。

为了充分利用生物监测的数据,必须把测量数据和与生物标记相关的任一DNEL 或外部 DNEL 进行比较。其中,在与外部 DNEL 比较的情况下,必须有数据表明生物标志物的水平和外部剂量度量之间的关系。以生物标志物和外部剂量度量之间关系为基础,应明确说明其毒代动力学性质(例如吸收百分比)。

4. 不确定性和统计学

与职业暴露评价相关的不确定性有很多种,它们是:

- 测量的不确定性(来源于采样方法);
- 测量结果的选择;
- 模拟结果的不确定性;
- 评价的不确定性。

如果忽略不确定性或变化性的因素,或者没有给出对最终评估可能产生的影响,都将影响评估精度和准确度。所有这些不确定性和可变性,需要与相关风险评估过程中毒理学数据的不确定性一起考虑。这些不确定性,在某些情况下可以通过使用一个更保守的估算值进行补充,特别是当它们与暴露现场数据的代表性和适当性有关的时候。

在暴露信息并入暴露评估之前,需要仔细评估其数据质量和适用性。这种评估通常使用职业卫生的专业知识,而不是简单地应用公约或直接使用统计方法进行。例如,计算通常需要考虑该信息被收集的条件,以确定该信息的代表性,因此在暴露过程中将对相关性和权重进行评估。工作流程出错时收集的数据可能不代表日常操作,但在一定条件下也可以得到其他可借鉴的结论。另外,大量从工厂的常规操作上收集的物质信息,几乎完全能代表相同物质的许多下游用途。在对实测数据进行统计分析时,需要用到统计相关的专业知识。对于暴露的估计,需要比较常规 DNELs 或 DMELs 与最高可能暴露浓度。在测定数据中能代表最高暴露的数据取决于测量本身,通常是暴露分布的较高水平部分。

评价亚组之间的可能区别,一方面可用来防止低估风险(如果亚组的较高暴露被其他亚组的较低暴露水平掩盖),另一方面可用来防止在操作条件和风险管理措施要求上的过度保守(例如,如果某些风险管理措施旨在针对高暴露的亚组,而不是针对总的暴露群体)。基于这样的分析,相关管理人员可以选择为高暴露组建立一个单独的暴露现场。

如果管理人员打算立足于一组测量数据进行暴露评估,应考虑一些一般性的规则,选择来自暴露分布的代表值时(对于可能的最高的暴露情况)需要判断:

评估暴露数据是否足以反映暴露场景,如果是,则选择合适的百分位数。

- 建议选择特定暴露场景条件下全部暴露分布的 90%。
- 在特殊的条件下,其他百分位数也可能适用。

例如,如果所测量的数据集仅代表最高暴露,但被应用于表征更广范围的情况,并在暴露的实际百分数超过选定值但远低于 25%,则可以适当使用暴露测量值的 75%。

　　另一种情况,当测量值是一个意义明确、高质量的数据时,也可使用更低的百分比,这些数据一般较均一,分布范围很窄,其特点是风险特性比率明显低于 1,并且充分代表了暴露场景中描述的操作条件和风险管理措施。

　　作为化学品安全评价中的职业暴露评价,不推荐使用测量数据的 50% 或者中值。

5. 不同情况下的暴露评估

　　例如,欧洲职业现场评价给出的一个例子,暴露场景是"含有物质 X 的涂料滚动涂刷",该涂料在整个欧洲都有使用,所有季节的室内和室外同时适用。含有涂料物质 X 可以是含量相对高的 X 或相对较低的 X(例如 5%～30%),暴露场景也应该包括所有的可能性。在方案中的高暴露情况,是南欧的工人在夏天室内使用含 X 30% 的涂料。在欧洲测得的有效数据中没有涂料 X 含量、测量地区或者测量温度的任何信息。在这种情况下,暴露分布的高百分位数(例如,第 90 百分位)应作为一个合理的最高暴露情况。然而,对于使用含 30% X 涂料的南非地区工人,有一组非常特殊的数据,这种场景必须包括较低百分数值(例如第 75 个百分位数)的较低暴露情况(所用的涂料含较低量的 X、测量过程中温度较低)。全部有效数据、处理过程中所做的假设和数据解释都需要在信息收集评价表中被证明并记录下来。

　　另一个通常不推荐的参数是数据集的最大值,因为工作人员通常暴露在一个对数分布的环境中,一般不可能在很高浓度的环境下持续暴露。很多数据集都有一或两个很高的值,有时候会有最大值。这些最大值不能合理地代表最高暴露环境,通常会高估风险。当然,如果一组典型数据的最大值明显低于 DNEL,则可以用得到的最大值来对安全性结论进行评估。这个最大值通常与代表了特殊亚组的高暴露值有关,这可以用于证明特殊的暴露场景。

6.2.6　急性暴露

　　一些物质发生接触暴露可能诱发急性健康效应,如果还存在高剂量暴露的可能,则应该建立急性 DNEL。同样,建立急性暴露限值需要高质量和可靠的数据进行支持。

　　现在并没有特别的定义用于说明急性暴露和急性 DNEL。如果是持续很短的时间(几秒到几分钟),这种评估主要从在线直读仪器上反映出来,另一方面,如果急性暴露时间接近于全程监测暴露的结果时,则不用再去区分急性暴露与全程暴露情况的差异。呼吸暴露考察的最少平均暴露时间为 15 min,这与通常所谓的短期暴露时间 15 min 是一样的(EC2000),测量数据文档应包含采样时间。

急性暴露评估与常规的 8 h 暴露评估不同,这种短期暴露评估应该考虑急性效应种类。例如,某些物质不能超过一定的剂量值,超过就会导致死亡。这需要了解呼吸暴露的最高限值。某些情况下,如果急性暴露的发生比较短暂,不严重,并且不是长期效应的首要影响,则可以忽略,继续采用此剂量。通常急性效应是在暴露后立刻发生的,或暴露后经过一段时间,甚至在多次时断时续的暴露后发生的,则可以将总剂量的一定比例(如 95%)作为合理的最高暴露剂量,在此剂量下,只会产生不甚严重的可恢复的健康效应。

在同样条件下,相比长时间总的暴露情况,急性暴露测量数据有很强的可变性。急性暴露数值也彼此相关,参数之间会有很大相关性变化。基于这些认识,有研究计算了急性暴露评估与全程暴露评估之间的对比关系[112],同样的情况,对于 15 min 的暴露数据,95% 的数值大致是 90% 数值的两倍,是 75% 数值的四倍。

急性暴露检测通常是针对风险度很高的环境。在这种情况下,也需要与常规监测同样的测量过程,当很难准确预估高暴露释放时间,且偶尔出现急性暴露时,则需要更多的测量数据支持。通常对于估计急性暴露分布的 95% 量值时,最少需要做 20 个短期暴露监测。当暴露情况的不确定性很高,或最高暴露剂量几乎与短期暴露限值接近时,则需要考虑设计更高数量的测量工作。

职业暴露限值主要根据 8 h 暴露进行计算,这是因为慢性健康效应主要关注暴露的气溶胶物质。因此,在大多数工作环境下,只用 8 h 轮换的暴露数据或估计值,而同样在某些情况下,需要关注急性暴露水平,这就需要使用全程时间监测数据计算急性暴露数据。这种统计推算可用于不严重及短期急性效应数据推算,而不适用于非常严重的效应推算,比如短期暴露致死剂量。

从全程时间监测数据推算急性暴露剂量基于大多数暴露分布呈正态分布,几何平均(GM)和几何标准差(GSDs)分布与不同平均时间段相关[112]。可通过对数正态分布的几何平均数和标准差计算百分位数,因此百分位数分布与不同的平均时间段相关。对于全程时间监测数据或急性暴露数据,百分位数作为合理的最高暴露浓度不都是一个固定的百分比,基于(不确定性)的数据和估计的认为合适的情况下,可以使用评估从第 75 到第 90 百分位数作为全程监测暴露数据的评估数据,由于暴露本身的严重性,急性暴露估计可以采用一个相对较高的百分位数。

合理的急性暴露最高值可以从全程监测数据中用一个倍增因子进行换算。这个因子取决于合理的最高暴露值的保守性要求,比如将急性暴露中的第多少百分位数作为合理的最高可能暴露值。这也取决于评估最高暴露值时的百分位数及可变性。表 6.2 是根据 Kumagai 和 Matsunaga 方程从全程监测数据推算短期 15 分钟暴露最大值的例子[112]。

表 6.2　利用倍增因子从全程监测数据中确定合理的急性暴露最高值

暴露情况	每天全程监测数据中 最高暴露值＝第 75 百分位		每天全程监测数据中 最高暴露值＝第 90 百分位	
急性(15 min 的 平均估计量)	95 百分位点	99 百分位点	95 百分位点	99 百分位点
低可变性(默认值)	4	20	2	6
高可变性	6	40	1.5	10

　　总之,安全性评价是建立在现场监测数据的基础上进行的,既需要专业性很强的统计分析知识,也需要结合不同监测现场的具体条件进行案例分析评价。

第7章 总结与展望

尽管纳米技术是工业领域一个相对较新的分支,但是已有大量产品问世,据估计,市场上有 400 多种使用纳米材料的消费品。

纳米技术主要应用于以下领域:

■ 复合材料——提高产品的耐磨性、硬度、绝缘性,用于涂料可提高涂层的抗污性、耐受性、附着力、抗菌性等。

■ 健康保健——应用于新药、活性剂、药物控释系统、口服疫苗、组织工程学以及生物相容性材料。

■ 能量转换与使用——用于低损耗的能量存储,提高能量转化效率,包括新一代光电管、更经济的节能灯、压缩的燃料电池。

■ 汽车、航天产业——更加强劲的材料、传感器优化引擎使用、燃料添加剂、防刮痕材料、防尘涂料等。

■ 化学工业——催化剂、无胶键合技术、多功能高效制陶艺术、适用于材料表面功能化和成型,如防腐蚀剂、自动清洁表面、防静电、功能层等。

■ 电子信息产业——光学/光电子元件包括激光、高密度存储器、袖珍型电子图书馆、超快速的超薄型电脑。

随着纳米材料的广泛应用,其安全性日益引起多领域专家的关注,针对纳米毒理学与安全性评价这两个领域,生产场所纳米颗粒暴露释放研究是连接两个研究领域的纽带。随着现场暴露的深入开展,现场评价步骤、方案逐渐规范,不同暴露现场能够进行横向对比,则可以正确认识纳米材料生产现场的安全性。现场暴露与防护关系着产业工人的安全与健康,提高对现场暴露风险的正确认识将可以塑造一个可期待的美好纳米未来世界。

人类总是暴露于高度变化的大气环境,颗粒物数量浓度低则在几百,高则几百万(每立方厘米空气)。这些颗粒物来源于多种自然以及人为活动,如森林火灾、交通、火源等。由这些活动产生的纳米尺度颗粒物都属于纳米颗粒范畴。然而,它们的形态和化学成分与人造纳米颗粒又有所不同。为了更好地评估纳米材料的暴露释放行为,我们需要将其与其他来源的颗粒进行区分。在工业场所中,需要鉴定区分背景空气中的纳米颗粒,如源于供热机组、叉车、真空清洁器等的纳米颗粒。室外来源同样也要考虑。

在纳米安全逐渐形成与发展的路上可能会遇到如下挑战:测量参数的不确定性(如颗粒大小、数量、质量、表面积等);监测方法一致性问题(如监测策略、校准方案、风险评估模型等);详细职业暴露评估的繁琐高花费以及需要精细的分析和设计。此外,高效评估方法,如分组或分层次的暴露评估研究方案对现场研究可以起到高效和全面的风险评估效果。面对越来越多的纳米材料应用,需要寻找更加高效和完善的解决方案以完成纳米材料职业安全评价工作,为纳米科技的可持续发展保驾护航。

附录 1　国内纳米安全与暴露现场监测文献汇编

1. He, X., Zhang, Z. Y., Liu, J. S., Ma, Y. H., Zhang, P., Li, Y. Y., Wu, Z. Q., Zhao, Y. L., Chai, Z. F. Quantifying the biodistribution of nanoparticles. Nat. Nanotechnol., 2011, 6: 755-755.

2. Chen, C. Y., Li, Y. F., Qu, Y., Chai, Z. F., Zhao, Y. L. Advanced nuclear analytical and related techniques for the growing challenges of nanotoxicology. Chem. Soc. Rev., 2013, 42(21): 8266-8303.

3. Liu, Y., Zhao, Y. L., Sun, B. Y., Chen C. Y. Understanding the toxicity of carbon nanotubes. Acc. Chem. Res, 2013, 46(3): 702-713.

4. Zhu, M. T., Nie, G. J., Meng, H., Xia, T., Nel, A., Zhao, Y. L. Physicochemical properties determine nanomaterial cellular uptake, transport and fate. Acc. Chem. Res., 2013, 46(3): 622-631.

5. Wang, B., He, X., Zhang, Z. Y., Zhao, Y. L., Feng, W. Y. Metabolism of nanomaterials in vivo: blood circulation and organ clearance. Acc. Chem. Res., 2013, 46(3): 761-769.

6. Nel, A., Zhao, Y. L., Mädler, L. Environmental health and safety considerations for nanotechnology. Acc. Chem. Res., 2013, 46(3): 605-606.

7. 陈田, 甄森, 贾光. 纳米颗粒的职业风险管理. 中华预防医学杂志, 2010, 44(9): 828-830.

8. Zhao, F., Zhao, Y., Liu, Y., Chang, X. L., Chen, C. Y., Zhao, Y. L. Cellular uptake, intracellular trafficking, and cytotoxicity of nanomaterials. Small, 2011, 7(10): 1322-1337.

9. Zhao, F., Meng, H., Yan, L., Wang, B., Zhao, Y. L. Nanosurface chemistry and dose govern the bioaccumulation and toxicity of carbon nanotubes, metal nanomaterials and quantum dots in vivo. Sci. Bull., 2015, 60(1): 3-20.

10. 徐莺莺, 林晓影, 陈春英. 影响纳米材料毒性的关键因素. 科学通报, 2013, 58(24): 2466-2478.

11. 王越, 王鹏, 陈春英, 赵宇亮. 碳纳米管呼吸系统毒性作用机制及其影响因素的研究进展. 科学通报, 2013, 58(21): 2007-2020.

12. 吴添舒, 唐萌. 人造纳米颗粒呼吸系统毒性及生物效应的研究进展. 科学通报, 2015, 60(8): 727-740.

13. 熊丽林,吴添舒,唐萌. 大气纳米颗粒物对人体健康效应的研究进展. 中华预防医学杂志,2015,49(9):88-91.

14. Zhen, S., Qian, Q., Jia, G., Zhang, J., Chen, C. Y., Wei, Y. J. A panel study for cardiopulmonary effects produced by occupational exposure to inhalable titanium dioxide. J. Occup. Environ. Med., 2012, 54(11): 1389-1394.

15. 甄森,张济,马衍辉,张宁,刘岚铮,王天成,陈春英,周敬文,李新伟,钱琴,吕艳朋,林少倩,贾光. 车间二氧化钛接触对职业人群氧化应激水平影响的定群研究. 中华预防医学杂志,2010,44(9):775-779.

16. Chen, R., Shi, X. F., Bai, R., Rang, W. Q., Huo, L. L., Zhao, L., Long, D. X., Pui, D. Y. H., Chen, C. Y. Airborne nanoparticle pollution in a wire electrical discharge machining workshop and potential health risks. Aerosol Air Qual. Res., 2015, 15(1): 284-294.

17. Jing, H., Li, Y. F., Zhao. J. T., Li. B., Sun, J. L. Wide-range particle characterization and elemental concentration in Beijing aerosol during the 2013 spring festival. Environ. Pollut., 2014, 192: 204-211.

18. Ge, C. C., Du, J. F., Zhao, L. N., Wang, L. M., Liu, Y., Li, D. H., Yang, Y. L., Zhou, R. H., Zhao, Y. L., Chai, Z. F., Chen, C. Y. Binding of blood proteins to carbon nanotubes reduces cytotoxicity. Proc. Natl. Acad. Sci. USA, 2011, 108(41): 16968-16973.

19. Ge, C. C., Li, Y., Yin, J. J., Liu, Y., Wang, L. M., Zhao, Y. L., Chen, C. Y. The contributions of metal impurities and tube structure to the toxicity of carbon nanotube materials. NPG Asia Mater., 2012, 4: e32.

20. Ge, C. C., Meng, L., Xu, L. G., Bai, R., Du, J. F., Zhang, L. L., Li, Y., Chang, Y. Z., Zhao, Y. L., Chen, C. Y. Acute pulmonary and moderate cardiovascular responses of spontaneously hypertensive rats after exposure to single-wall carbon nanotubes. Nanotoxicology, 2012, 6(5): 526-542.

21. Chen, R., Zhang, L. L, Ge, C. C., Tseng, M., Bai, R., Qu, Y., Beer, C., Autrup, H., Chen, C. Y. Subchronic toxicity and cardiovascular responses in spontaneously hypertensive rats after exposure to multiwalled carbon nanotubes by intratracheal instillation. Chem. Res. Toxicol., 2015, 28(3): 440-450.

22. Wang, P., Wang, Y., Nie, X., Céline Braini, Bai R., Chen C. Y. Multiwall carbon nanotubes directly promote fibroblast-myofibroblast and epithelial-mesenchymal transitions through the activation of the TGF-β/Smad signaling

pathway. Small, 2015; 11(4):446-455.

23. Wang, P. , Nie, X. , Wang, Y. , Li, Y. , Ge, C. C. , Zhang, L. , Wang, L. , Bai, R. , Chen, Z. , Zhao, Y. L. , Chen, C. Y. Multiwall carbon nanotubes mediate macrophage activation and promote pulmonary fibrosis through TGF-β/Smad signaling pathway. Small, 2013, 9(22):3799-3811.

24. Chen, T. , Nie, H. Y. , Gao, X. , Yang, J. L. , Pu, J. , Chen, Z. J. , Cui, X. X. , Wang, Y. , Wang, H. F. , Jia, G. Epithelial-mesenchymal transition involved in pulmonary fibrosis induced by multi-walled carbon nanotubes via TGF-beta/Smad signaling pathway. Toxicol. Lett. , 2014, 226(2):150-162.

25. Wang, X. , Guo, J. , Chen, T. , Nie, H. Y. , Wang, H. F. , Zang, J. J. , Cui, X. X. , Jia, G. Multi-walled carbon nanotubes induce apoptosis via mitochondrial pathway and scavenger receptor. Toxicol. *In Vitro*, 2012, 26(6): 799-806.

26. Meng, L. , Chen, R. , Jiang, A. H. , Wang, L. M. , Wang, P. , Li, C. Z. , Bai, R. , Zhao, Y. L. , Autrup, H. , Chen, C. Y. Short multiwall carbon nanotubes promote neuronal differentiation of PC12 cells *via* up-regulation of the neurotrophin signaling pathway. Small, 2013, 9(9-10):1786-1798.

27. Meng, L. , Jiang, A. H. , Chen, R. , Li, C. Z. , Wang, L. M. , Qu, Y. , Wang, P. , Zhao, Y. L. , Chen, C. Y. Inhibitory effects of multiwall carbon nanotubes with high iron impurity on viability and neuronal differentiation in cultured PC12 cells. Toxicology, 2013, 313(1):49-58.

28. Jia, G. , Wang, H. F. , Yan, L. , Wang, X. , Pei, R. J. , Yan, T. , Zhao, Y. L. , Guo, X. B. Cytotoxicity of carbon nanomaterials: Single-wall nanotube, multi-wall nanotube, and fullerene. Environ. Sci. Technol. , 2005, 39(5): 1378-1383.

29. Chen, H. Q. , Wang, B. , Gao, D. , Guan, M. , Zheng, L. N. , Ouyang, H. , Chai, Z. F. , Zhao, Y. L. , Feng, W. Y. Broad-spectrum antibacterial activity of carbon nanotubes to human gut bacteria. Small, 2013, 9 (16): 2735-2746.

30. Zhao, Y. L. , Wu, Q. L. , Li, Y. P. , Nouara, A. , Jia, R. H. , Wang, D. Y. In vivo translocation and toxicity of multi-walled carbon nanotubes are regulated by microRNAs. Nanoscale, 2014, 6(8):4275-4284.

31. Chen, Z. Y. , Liu, Y. , Sun, B. Y. , Li, H. , Dong, J. Q. , Zhang, L. J. , Wang, L. M. , Wang, P. , Zhao, Y. L. , Chen, C. Y. Polyhydroxylated metallofullerenols stimulate IL-1 secretion of macrophage through TLRs/MyD88/

NF-κB pathway and NLRP3 inflammasome activation. Small, 2014, 10(12): 2362-2372.

32. Pang, C. F. , Brunelli, A. , Zhu, C. H. , Hristozov, D. , Liu, Y. , Semenzin, E. , Wang, W. W. , Tao, W. Q. , Liang, J. N. , Marcomini, A. , Chen, C. Y. , Zhao, B. Demonstrating approaches to chemically modify the surface of Ag nanoparticles in order to influence their cytotoxicity and biodistribution after single dose acute intravenous administration. Nanotoxicology, 2015, DOI: 10.3109/17435390.2015.1024295.

33. Wang, L. M. , Zhang, T. L. , Li, P. Y. , Huang, W. X. , Tang, J. L. , Wang, P. Y. , Liu, J. , Yuan, Q. X. , Bai, R. , Li, B. , Zhang, K. Zhao, Y. L. , Chen, C. Y. Use of synchrotron radiation-analytical techniques to reveal chemical origin of silver-nanoparticle cytotoxicity. ACS Nano, 2015, 23, 9(6): 6532-6547.

34. Huo, L. L. , Chen, R. Zhao, L. Shi, X. F. , Bai, R. , Long, D. X. , Chen, F. , Zhao, Y. L. , Chang, Y. Z. , Chen, C. Y. Silver nanoparticles activate endoplasmic reticulum stress signaling pathway in cell and mouse models: The role in toxicity evaluation. Biomaterials. 2015, 61, 307-315.

35. Jiang, X. M. , Teodora Miclaus, Wang, L. M. , Rasmus Foldbjerg, Duncan S. Sutherland, Herman Autrup, Chen C. Y. , Christiane Beer. Fast intracellular dissolution and persistent cellular uptake of silver nanoparticles in CHO-K1 cells: implication for cytotoxicity. Nanotoxicology, 2015, 9 (2): 181-189.

36. Wang, L. M. , Li, J. Y. , Pan, J. , Jiang, X. M. , Ji, Y. L. , Li, Y. F. , Qu, Y. , Zhao, Y. L. , Wu, X. C. , Chen, C. Y. Revealing the binding structure of the protein corona on gold nanorods using synchrotron radiation-based techniques: Understanding the reduced damage in cell membranes. J. Am. Chem. Soc. , 2013, 135(46):17359-17368.

37. Wang, L. M. , Jiang, X. M. , Ji, Y. L. , Bai, R. , Zhao, Y. L. , Wu, X. C. , Chen, C. Y. Surface chemistry of gold nanorods: origin of cell membrane damage and cytotoxicity. Nanoscale,2013, 5(18):8384-8391.

38. Qiu, Y. , Liu, Y. , Wang, L. M. , Xu, L. G. , Bai, R. , Ji, Y. L. , Wu, X. C. , Zhao, Y. L. , Li, Y. F. , Chen, C. Y. Surface chemistry and aspect ratio mediated cellular uptake of Au nanorods. Biomaterials, 2010, 31 (30): 7606-7619.

39. Zhu, M. T. , Li, Y. Y. , Shi, J. , Feng, W. Y. , Nie, G. J. , Zhao, Y.

L. Cellular responses to nanomaterials: Exosomes as extrapulmonary signaling conveyors for nanoparticle-induced systemic immune activation. Small, 2012, 8 (3): 404-412.

40. Zhu, M. T., Tian, X., Song, X., Li, Y. Y., Tian, Y. H., Zhao, Y. L., Nie, G. J. Nanoparticle-induced exosomes target antigen-presenting cells to initiate Th1-type immune activation. Small, 2012, 8(18): 2841-2848.

41. Zhu, M. T., Wang, B., Wang, Y., Yuan, L., Wang, H. J., Wang, M., Ouyang, H., Chai, Z. F., Feng, W. Y., Zhao, Y. L. Endothelial dysfunction and inflammation induced by iron oxide nanoparticle exposure: Risk factors for early atherosclerosis. Toxicol. Lett., 2011, 203(2):162-171.

42. Wang, Y., Wang, B., Zhu, M. T., Li, M., Wang, H. J., Wang, M., Ouyang, H., Chai, Z. F., Feng, W. Y., Zhao, Y. L. Microglial activation, recruitment and phagocytosis as linked phenomena in ferric oxide nanoparticle exposure. Toxicol. Lett., 2011, 205(1):26-37.

43. Qu, Y., Li, W., Zhou, Y., Liu, X., Zhang, L., Wang, L., Li, Y., Iida, A., Tang, Z., Zhao, Y., Chai, Z., Chen,C. Full assessment of fate and physiological behavior of quantum dots utilizing caenorhabditis elegans as a model organism. Nano Lett., 2011, 11(8): 3174-3183.

44. Li, Y. Y., Zhou, Y. L., Wang, H. Y., Perrett, S., Zhao, Y. L., Tang, Z. Y., Nie, G. J. Chirality of glutathione surface coating affects the cytotoxicity of quantum dots. Angew. Chem. Int. Ed. Engl., 2011, 50 (26): 5860-5864.

45. Liu, Y. X., Wang, P., Wang, Y., Zhu, Z. N., Lao, F., Liu, X. F., Cong, W. S., Chen, C. Y., Gao, Y., Liu, Y. The influence on cell cycle and cell division by various cadmium-containing quantum dots. Small, 2013, 9(14): 2440-2451.

46. Zhang, W. D., Wang, C., Li, Z. J., Lu, Z. Z., Li, Y. Y., Yin, J. J., Zhou, Y. T., Gao, X. F., Fang, Y., Nie, G. J., Zhao, Y. L. Unraveling stress-induced toxicity properties of graphene oxide and the underlying mechanism. Adv. Mater., 2012, 24(39): 5391-5397.

47. Zhang, W. D., Sun, B. Y., Zhang, L. Z., Zhao, B. L., Nie, G. J., Zhao, Y. L. Biosafety assessment of Gd@C_{82}(OH)$_{22}$ nanoparticles on Caenorhabditiselegans. Nanoscale, 2011, 3(6): 2636-2641.

48. Cong. W. S., Wang, P., Qu, Y., Tang, J. L., Bai, R., Zhao, Y. L., Chen, C. Y., Bi, X. L. Evaluation of the influence of fullerenol on aging and

stress resistance using Caenorhabditis elegans. Biomaterials, 2015, 42: 78-86.

49. Chen, R., Huo, L. L., Shi, X. F., Bai, R., Zhang, Z. J., Zhao, Y. L., Chang, Y. Z., Chen, C. Y. Endoplasmic reticulum stress induced by zinc oxide nanoparticles is an earlier biomarker for nanotoxicological evaluation. ACS Nano, 2014, 8(3): 2562-2574.

50. Li, J. X., Chang, X. L., Chen, X. X., Gu, Z. J., Zhao, F., Chai, Z. F., Zhao, Y. L. Toxicity of inorganic nanomaterials in biomedical imaging. Biotechnol. Adv., 2014, 32(4): 727-743.

51. Zuo, G. H., Kang, S. G., Xiu, P., Zhao, Y. L., Zhou, R. H. Interactions between proteins and carbon-based nanoparticles: exploring the origin of nanotoxicity at molecular level. Small, 2013, 9(9-10):1546-1556.

52. Chen, X. X., Cheng, B., Yang, Y. X., Cao, A. N., Liu, J. H., Du, L. J., Liu, Y. F., Zhao, Y. L., Wang, H. F. Characterization and preliminary toxicity assay of nano-titanium dioxide additive in sugar-coated chewing gum. Small, 2013, 9(9-10): 1765-1774.

53. Zhang, L. L., Bai, R., Li, B., Ge, C. C., Du, J. F., Liu, Y., Le Guyader, L., Zhao, Y. L., Wu, Y., He, S. D., Ma, Y. M., Chen, C. Y. Rutile TiO_2 particles exert size and surface coating dependent retention and lesions on the murine brain. Toxicol. Lett., 2011, 207(1): 73-81.

54. Zhang, X. Q., Yin, L. H., Tang, M., Pu, Y. P. ZnO, TiO_2, SiO_2, and Al_2O_3 nanoparticles-induced toxic effects on human fetal lung fibroblasts. Biomed. Environ. Sci., 2011, 24(6): 661-669.

55. Tian, X., Zhu, M. T., Du, L. B., Wang, J., Fan, Z. L., Liu, J., Zhao, Y. L., Nie, G. J. Intrauterine inflammation increases materno-fetal transfer of gold nanoparticles in a size-dependent manner in murine pregnancy. Small, 2013, 9: 2432-2439.

56. Yang, H., Sun, C. J., Fan, Z. L., Tian, X., Yan, L., Du, L. B., Liu, Y., Chen, C. Y., Liang, X. J., Anderson, G. J., Keelan, J. A., Zhao, Y. L., Nie, G. J. Effects of gestational age and surface modification on materno-fetal transfer of nanoparticles in murine pregnancy. Sci. Rep., 2012, 2: 847.

57. Lv, X. F., Liu, Y., Kong, X. J., Lobie, P. E., Chen, C. Y., Zhu, T. Nanotoxicity: A growing need for study in the endocrine system. Small, 2013, 9(9-10): 1654-1671.

58. He, X., Zhang, H. F., Ma, Y. H., Bai, W., Zhang, Z. Y., Lu, K., Ding, Y. Y., Zhao, Y. L., Chai, Z. F. Lung deposition and extrapulmo-

nary translocation of nano-ceria after intratracheal instillation. Nanotechnology, 2010, 21(28): 285103.

59. He, X. , Kuang, Y. , Li, Y. Y. , Zhang, H. F. , Ma, Y. H. , Bai, W. , Zhang, Z. Y. , Wu, Z. Q. , Zhao, Y. L. , Chai, Z. F. Changing exposure media can reverse the cytotoxicity of ceria nanoparticles for Escherichia coli. Nanotoxicology, 2012, 6(3): 233-240.

60. Ma, Y. H. , He, X. , Zhang, P. , Zhang, Z. Y. , Guo, Z. , Tai, R. Z. , Xu, Z. J. , Zhang, L. J. , Ding, Y. Y. , Zhao, Y. L. , Chai, Z. F. Phytotoxicity and biotransformation of La_2O_3 nanoparticles in a terrestrial plant cucumber (Cucumis sativus). Nanotoxicology, 2011, 5(4):743-753.

61. Ma, Y. H. , Kuang, L. L. , He, X. , Bai, W. , Ding, Y. Y. , Zhang, Z. Y. , Zhao, Y. L. , Chai, Z. F. Effects of rare earth oxide nanoparticles on root elongation of plants. Chemosphere, 2010, 78(3):273-279.

62. Yan, L. , Zhao, F. , Li, S. F. , Hu, Z. B. , Zhao, Y. L. Low-toxic and safe nanomaterials by surface-chemical design, carbon nanotubes, fullerenes, metallofullerenes, and graphenes. Nanoscale, 2011, 3(2): 362-382.

63. Yan, L. , Gu, Z. J. , Zhao, Y. L. Chemical mechanisms of the toxicological properties of nanomaterials: generation of intracellular reactive oxygen species. Chem. Asian J. , 2013, 8: 2342-2353.

1. 定量纳米材料生物分布
Quantifying the biodistribution of nanoparticles

Subject terms: Nanoparticles Environmental, health and safety issues

To the Editor

Yamashita et al. (Nature Nanotech. 6, 321-328; 2011) report that silica and titanium dioxide (TiO$_2$) nanoparticles with diameters of 70 nm and 35 nm, respectively, can cross the placental barrier in pregnant mice. Using transmission electron microscopy (TEM), the researchers claim that nanoparticles are found in the liver and brain of the fetus. Although TEM is useful for the qualitative examination of nanoparticles, it is not sensitive enough for studying the transplacental transport of TiO$_2$ nanoparticles.

Assuming that the concentration of TiO$_2$ nanoparticles in the fetal liver is one nanogram per gram of liver (the density of liver is approximately 1. 1 g cm^{-3}) and that the mass of a 35 nm TiO$_2$ particle is approximately 1×10^{-16} g (the density of rutile-TiO$_2$ is 4. 3 g cm^{-3}), on average, only one nanoparticle can theoretically be found in a 1 mm^2 section of liver tissue (an ultrathin section usually has a thickness of less than 100 nm). The TEM images collected by Yamashita et al. showed a dark electron-dense spot in a field size of $\sim$5 μm $\times$ 5 μm. Based on our estimation, on average, tens of thousands of such images need to be examined to find one TiO$_2$ nanoparticle. This means that the TEM results cannot firmly prove that nanoparticles were present in the fetal liver and brain, unless the concentration of nanoparticles in the fetal liver is several orders of magnitude higher than the hypothetical value of one nanogram per gram.

In conclusion, more suitable quantitative methods should be used to study the biodistribution of nanoparticles in pregnant mice.

Nat. Nanotechnol., 2011, 6(12):755.

2. 先进的核分析技术迎接纳米毒理学日益增长的挑战
Advanced nuclear analytical and related techniques for the growing challenges of nanotoxicology

Abstract: Manufactured nanomaterials with novel physicochemical properties are an important basis for nanosciences and related technologies. Nanotoxicology, aiming to understand the principles of interactions at the nano-bio interface and the relationship between the physicochemical properties of nanomaterials and their toxicological profiles, has become a new frontier in nanoscience. Nearly one decade of nanotoxicology research has shown that the interactions between nano-materials and proteins, cells, animals, humans and the environment as well as the underlying mechanisms of toxicity for nanomaterials are remarkably compli-cated, requiring dedicated analytical methodology and tools. Because of their advantages of absolute quantification, high sensitivity, excellent accuracy and precision, low matrix effects and non-destructiveness, nuclear analytical tech-niques have been playing important roles in the study of nanotoxicology. A sys-tematic summary and comprehensive review of the advanced nuclear analytical and related techniques in nanotoxicology is greatly needed. In this review article, we present a comprehensive overview of nuclear analytical techniques applied to the physicochemical characterization of nanomaterials, structural analysis of bio-nano interactions, visualization of nanomaterials in vitro, quantification of bio-distribution, bio-accumulation, and transformation of nanomaterials in vivo. As important complementary tools, optical imaging technologies are also highlighted. Future directions regarding advanced nuclear analytical approaches for nanotoxi-cology are also discussed. The rapid development of advanced light source-based techniques will enable new high-throughput screening techniques and provide high sensitivity with low detection limits, which are required for the distribution, imaging, and structural analysis of nanomaterials, and the molecular information of biomarkers for all aspects of nanotoxicology.

Chem. Soc. Rev., 2013, 42(21): 8266-8303.

3. 理解碳纳米管毒性
Understanding the toxicity of carbon nanotubes

Abstract: Because of their unique physical, chemical, electrical, and mechanical properties, carbon nanotubes (CNTs) have attracted a great deal of research interest and have many potential applications. As large-scale production and application of CNTs increases, the general population is more likely to be exposed to CNTs either directly or indirectly, which has prompted considerable attention about human health and safety issues related to CNTs. Although considerable experimental data related to CNT toxicity at the molecular, cellular, and whole animal levels have been published, the results are often conflicting. Therefore, a systematic understanding of CNT toxicity is needed but has not yet been developed.

In this Account, we highlight recent investigations into the basis of CNT toxicity carried out by our team and by other laboratories. We focus on several important factors that explain the disparities in the experimental results of nanotoxicity, such as impurities, amorphous carbon, surface charge, shape, length, agglomeration, and layer numbers. The exposure routes, including inhalation, intravenous injection, or dermal or oral exposure, can also influence the in vivo behavior and fate of CNTs. The underlying mechanisms of CNT toxicity include oxidative stress, inflammatory responses, malignant transformation, DNA damage and mutation (errors in chromosome number as well as disruption of the mitotic spindle), the formation of granulomas, and interstitial fibrosis. These findings provide useful insights for de novo design and safe application of carbon nanotubes and their risk assessment to human health.

To obtain reproducible and accurate results, researchers must establish standards and reliable detection methods, use standard CNT samples as a reference control, and study the impact of various factors systematically. In addition, researchers need to examine multiple types of CNTs, different cell lines and animal species, multidimensional evaluation methods, and exposure conditions. To make results comparable among different institutions and countries, researchers need to standardize choices in toxicity testing such as that of cell line, animal species, and exposure conditions. The knowledge presented here should lead to a better understanding of the key factors that can influence CNT toxicity so that their unwanted toxicity might be avoided.

Acc. Chem. Res., 2013, 46 (3): 702-713.

4. 理化性质决定纳米材料在细胞内的吸收，转运和代谢
Physicochemical properties determine nanomaterial cellular uptake, transport and fate

Abstract: Although a growing number of innovations have emerged in the fields of nanobiotechnology and nanomedicine, new engineered nanomaterials (ENMs) with novel physicochemical properties are posing novel challenges to understand the full spectrum of interactions at the nano-bio interface. Because these could include potentially hazardous interactions, researchers need a comprehensive understanding of toxicological properties of nanomaterials and their safer design. In depth research is needed to understand how nanomaterial properties influence bioavailability, transport, fate, cellular uptake, and catalysis of injurious biological responses. Toxicity of ENMs differ with their size and surface properties, and those connections hold true across a spectrum of in vitro to in vivo nano-bio interfaces. In addition, the in vitro results provide a basis for modeling the biokinetics and in vivo behavior of ENMs. Nonetheless, we must use caution in interpreting in vitro toxicity results too literally because of dosimetry differences between in vitro and in vivo systems as well the increased complexity of an in vivo environment. In this Account, we describe the impact of ENM physicochemical properties on cellular bioprocessing based on the research performed in our groups. Organic, inorganic, and hybrid ENMs can be produced in various sizes, shapes and surface modifications and a range of tunable compositions that can be dynamically modified under different biological and environmental conditions. Accordingly, we cover how ENM chemical properties such as hydrophobicity and hydrophilicity, material composition, surface functionalization and charge, dispersal state, and adsorption of proteins on the surface determine ENM cellular uptake, intracellular biotransformation, and bioelimination versus bioaccumulation. We review how physical properties such as size, aspect ratio, and surface area of ENMs influence the interactions of these materials with biological systems, thereby affecting their hazard potential. We discuss our actual experimental findings and show how these properties can be tuned to control the uptake, biotransformation, fate, and hazard of ENMs. This Account provides specific information about ENM biological behavior and safety issues. This research also assists the development of safer nanotherapeutics and guides the design of new materials that can execute novel functions at the nano-bio interface.

Acc. Chem. Res., 2013, 46(3): 622-631.

5. 纳米材料在体内的代谢：血液循环与器官清除
Metabolism of nanomaterials *in vivo*：Blood circulation and organ clearance

Abstract：Before researchers apply nanomaterials（NMs）in biomedicine, they need to understand the blood circulation and clearance profile of these materials in vivo. These qualities determine the balance between nanomaterial-induced activity and unwanted toxicity. NMs have heterogeneous characteristics：they combine the bulk properties of solids with the mobility of molecules, and their highly active contact interfaces exhibit diverse functionalities. Any new and unexpected circulation features and clearance patterns are of great concern in toxicological studies and pharmaceutical screens. A number of studies have reported that NMs can enter the bloodstream directly during their application or indirectly via inhalation, ingestion, and dermal exposure. Due to the small size of NMs, the blood can then transport them throughout the circulation and to many organs where they can be stored. In this Account, we discuss the blood circulation and organ clearance patterns of NMs in the lung, liver, and kidney. The circulation of NMs in bloodstream is critical for delivery of inhalable NMs to extrapulmonary organs, the delivery of injectable NMs, the dynamics of tissue redistribution, and the overall targeting of drug carriers to specific cells and organs. The lung, liver, and kidney are the major distribution sites and target organs for NMs exposure, and the clearance patterns of NMs in these organs are critical for understanding the in vivo fate of NMs. Current studies suggest that multiple factors control the circulation and organ clearance of NMs. The size, shape, surface charge, surface functional groups, and aspect ratio of NMs as well as tissue microstructures strongly influence the circulation of NMs in bloodstream, their site-specific extravasation, and their clearance profiles within organs. Therefore structure design and surface modification can improve biocompatibility, regulate the in vivo metabolism, and reduce the toxicity of NMs. The biophysicochemical interactions occurring between NMs and between NMs and the biological milieu after the introduction of NMs into living systems may further influence the blood circulation and clearance profiles of NMs. These interactions can alter properties such as agglomeration, phase transformations, dissolution, degradation, protein adsorption, and surface reactivity. The physicochemical properties of NMs change dynamically in vivo thereby making the metabolism of NMs complex and difficult to predict. The development of in situ, real-time, and quantitative techniques, in vitro assays, and the adaptation of physiologically-based pharmacoki-netic (PBPK) and quantitative structure-activity relationship (QNSAR) modeling for NMs will streamline future in vivo studies.

Acc. Chem. Res. , 2013 , 46(3):761-769.

6. 纳米科技的环境健康与安全相关考量
Environmental health and safety considerations for nanotechnology

Abstract: An important conceptual advance in nanotechnology environmental and health (nano-EHS) assessment has been the recognition that the dynamic physicochemical properties of engineered nanomaterials (ENMs) play a key role in their fate and transport, human and environmental exposure, and hazard generation. Thus, it is imperative to develop robust in vitro and in vivo safety assessment approaches that relate specific material properties to possible mechanisms of biological injury, pathophysiology of disease, dosimetry, and exposure of humans and environment life forms. This requires critical knowledge acquisition about the unique interactions of organic, inorganic, and hybrid ENMs, as well as the commercial nanocomposites and derivative materials at the nano/bio interface, including the use of this information to establish structure activity relationships (SARs) and risk reduction strategies. We have come to recognize that, because of the diverse and unique properties of ENMs, safe implementation of nanotechnology and the governance of nano-EHS is a multidisciplinary exercise that goes beyond traditional hazard, exposure, and risk assessment strategies. This requires cooperation between academia, industry, government, and the public to allow for the proper coordination of nano-EHS activities, rational decision-making tools, and the development of sustainable technology approaches. These processes could be accelerated by implementation of predictive toxicological approaches and rapid throughput screening platforms, as well as exploiting computational methods to assist in the establishment of quantitative SARs and safer-by-design approaches. While basic knowledge is being gathered, it is important to develop appropriate incremental regulatory approaches for safe nano-EHS implementation and advancement of materials to the marketplace with public acceptance and Support.

In this special issue, we have brought together the views of experts in a variety of nano-EHS fields to illustrate, through brief review of impactful personal research, the current state-of-the-art in these novel scientific areas. Examples of the major nano-EHS topics that are covered in this issue include (i) delineation of the mechanisms of biological/chemical injury at the nano/bio interface from the perspective of ENM physicochemical properties, including how those properties could be changed to develop potentially safer materials, (ii) use of ENM libraries for hazard assessment, establishment of nano-SARs, and development of predictive in vitro/in vivo toxicological approaches, (iii) assessment of the environmental impact of nanotechnology, from both the perspective of hazard assessment and utility toward environmental remediation, (iv) assessment of nanomaterial fate, transport, exposure, and bioaccumulation, (v) occupational safety assessment and performance of lifecycle analysis, (vi) risk assessment and formulation of the principles on which to base nano-EHS regulatory decision-making and governance, (vii) implementation of high-throughput screening, computational decision-making tools and the establishment of a nanoinformatics platform, and (viii) implementation of safer-by-design and "green nano" strategies.

All considered, the above advances demonstrate that knowledge gathering and implementation of safe nanotechnology approaches are making incremental advances and nano-EHS is now being regarded as integral to the development of a sustainable technology rather being pursued as a post hoc cleanup exercise. Equally important, we trust that this special issue will stimulate new research and breakthrough ideas in how to use this transformative technology toward the betterment of human and environmental safety while allowing the commercial enterprise to grow to the benefit of society. We also envisage that the knowledge gathering at the nano/bio interface will introduce new tools to treat human disease as well as to remediate the environment through multidisciplinary research between chemistry, nanomaterial science, medicine, biology, and environmental sciences.

Acc. Chem. Res. , 2013 , 46（3）: 605-606.

7. 纳米颗粒的职业风险管理

Occupational risk management of engineered nanoparticles

　　摘要：纳米技术、信息技术和生物技术被科学界称为 21 世纪科技发展的三大支柱，正如微米技术是 20 世纪科学技术的象征，21 世纪科学技术的象征是纳米技术。由于物质在纳米尺度($0.1\sim100$ nm, 1 nm$=10^{-9}$m)下有特殊性质，纳米技术几乎在各个领域都呈现出广阔的应用前景，人们在工作和生活中接触到纳米材料的机会也越来越多。但纳米技术有可能是一把双刃剑，其生物安全性问题也受到科学家的关注。2009 年 8 月发表在 *European Respiratory Journal* 的《暴露于纳米颗粒环境中可能造成胸腔积液、肺纤维化和肉芽肿》一文，引发了学术界的激烈讨论。纳米毒理学家对论文的结论提出质疑，认为它未能提供直接证据证明纳米颗粒就是"杀人凶手"；职业环境健康专家则认为，不论女工之死是否由纳米颗粒引起，改善工作环境、确保职业安全是当务之急。笔者认为，尽管目前纳米颗粒对人体的致病机制尚无明确报道，但已有动物实验提示，纳米颗粒能直接对生物体造成损伤。至少这一事件再次凸显了纳米技术职业风险管理的重要性，尤其对于那些长时间接触纳米颗粒的职业人群。纳米材料的职业接触者应包括涉及纳米材料的职业安全和健康工作者、研究人员、工人、生产商及普通纳米技术产品的使用者，他们是最先接触到纳米材料的人群。考虑到纳米技术如同 X 射线的发现一样，也有可能是一把双刃剑，在发展纳米技术的同时，也要关注职业人群的健康。笔者重点论述了有关纳米产业职业风险管理的理论框架，并且叙述了在未确定其危害情况下，可采取的相关预防原则及措施。

中华预防医学杂志，2010，44(9)：828-830.

8. 纳米材料的细胞摄取,胞内转运和细胞毒性
Cellular uptake, intracellular trafficking, and cytotoxicity of nanomaterials

Abstract: The interactions of nanoparticles with the soft surfaces of biological systems like cells play key roles in executing their biomedical functions and in toxicity. The discovery or design of new biomedical functions, or the prediction of the toxicological consequences of nanoparticles in vivo, first require knowledge of the interplay processes of the nanoparticles with the target cells. This article focusses on the cellular uptake, location and translocation, and any biological consequences, such as cytotoxicity, of the most widely studied and used nanoparticles, such as carbon-based nanoparticles, metallic nanoparticles, and quantum dots. The relevance of the size and shape, composition, charge, and surface chemistry of the nanoparticles in cells is considered. The intracellular uptake pathways of the nanoparticles and the cellular responses, with potential signaling pathways activated by nanoparticle interactions, are also discussed.

Keywords: nanoparticles; endocytosis; intracellular trafficking; cytotoxicity; signaling pathways

Small, *2011*, *7(10)*: *1322-1337*.

9. 纳米表面化学和剂量决定碳纳米管、金属纳米材料及量子点在体内的蓄积与毒性
Nanosurface chemistry and dose govern the bioaccumulation and toxicity of carbon nanotubes, metal nanomaterials and quantum dots *in vivo*

Abstract: The chemical and biological mechanisms of life processes mostly consist of multistep and programmed processes at nanoscale levels. Interestingly enough, cell, the basic functional unit and platform that maintains life processes, is composed of various organelles fulfilling sophisticated functions through the precise control on the biomolecules (e. g., proteins, phospholipid, nucleic acid and ions) in a spatial dimension of nanoscale sizes. Thus, understanding of the activities of manufactured nanoscale materials including their interaction with biological systems is of great significance in chemistry, materials science, life science, medicine, environmental science and toxicology. In this brief review, we summarized the recent advances in nanotoxicological chemistry through the dissection of pivotal factors (primarily focusing on dose and nanosurface chemistry) in determining nanomaterial-induced biological/toxic responses with particular emphasis on the nanomaterial bioaccumulation (and interaction organs or target organs) at intact animal level. Due to the volume of manufacture and material application, we deliberately discussed carbon nanotubes, metal/metal oxide nanomaterials and quantum dots, severing as representative material types to illustrate the impact of dose and nanosurface chemistry in these toxicological scenarios. Finally, we have also delineated the grand challenges in this field in a conceptual framework of nanotoxicological chemistry. It is noted that this review is a part of our persistent endeavor of building the systematic knowledge framework for toxicological properties of engineered nanomaterials.

Keywords: bioaccumulation; toxicity; targeted organs; carbon nanotubes; metal nanomaterials; quantum dots

Sci. Bull., 2015, 60(1): 3-20.

10. 影响纳米材料毒性的关键因素
Key factors influencing the toxicity of nanomaterials

摘要：随着纳米技术的发展，越来越多的纳米产品开始进入人们的日常生活，纳米材料的毒性因此成为人们日渐关注的问题。近年来，纳米材料毒性的研究取得了很大进展，包括体内和体外实验研究纳米材料与生物大分子、细胞、器官和组织的相互作用以及其引起的毒性。纳米材料通过诱导氧化应激和炎症反应等机制产生一系列毒性效应。纳米材料本身的物理化学性质对其毒性有决定性的影响，这些性质包括尺寸、形状、表面电荷、化学组成、表面修饰、金属杂质、团聚与分散性、降解性能以及"蛋白冠"的形成。阐明物化性质对纳米材料毒性的影响，对于纳米材料的合理设计和安全应用具有重要的意义。本文对影响纳米材料毒性的关键因素进行了总结和分析，对近年来纳米材料毒性效应的研究进展进行了综述。

关键词：纳米材料；纳米毒理学；物理化学性质；蛋白冠；氧化应激；炎症

科学通报，*2013*，*58（24）*：*2466-2478*.

11. 碳纳米管呼吸系统毒性作用机制及其影响因素的研究进展

Cellular and molecular mechanisms of pulmonary toxicity caused by carbon nanotubes with various physiochemical properties

　　摘要： 碳纳米管具有独特的力学、电学以及化学性质,使其能够在信息、光电、能源、传感、材料以及医疗等多个领域都有潜在的应用。与此同时,随着碳纳米管的广泛应用及其生产规模的日益扩大,碳纳米管的生物安全性也引起了越来越广泛的关注。近年来,许多研究人员从不同层次包括分子、细胞以及动物水平研究了碳纳米管的呼吸系统毒性,取得了大量的实验数据,然而许多研究结论并不一致,甚至相互矛盾,这可能与研究者所用碳纳米管的金属杂质种类及其含量、分散性、长度、直径等因素有关。本文从碳纳米管的结构和性质出发,阐述了近年来关于碳纳米管呼吸系统毒性及其细胞作用机制的研究进展,对可能影响碳纳米管细胞毒性的诸多因素进行了归纳和讨论。最后,我们对将来如何系统科学地研究和评价碳纳米管呼吸系统毒性作了展望。

　　关键词： 碳纳米管；纳米毒理学；肺毒性；毒性机制；理化性质

科学通报，2013，58(21)：2007-2020.

12. 人造纳米颗粒呼吸系统毒性及生物效应的研究进展

Research advances on the toxic effects of manufactured nanoparticles on the respiratory system

摘要：随着纳米技术在全球的迅猛发展，人造纳米颗粒已经广泛应用于生物医学领域，其生物安全性成为研究者的关注热点。由于呼吸道是人造纳米颗粒进入机体的主要途径之一，纳米颗粒对机体呼吸系统的毒性和生物效应的相关研究越来越多。本文介绍了人造纳米颗粒和纳米药物在治疗呼吸系统疾病中的应用，重点归纳了几种常见人造纳米颗粒对机体呼吸系统的毒性效应和可能的毒性作用机制，阐述了影响纳米颗粒毒性的几点因素，为今后人造纳米颗粒的研究和应用提供有价值的参考。

关键词：人造纳米颗粒；毒理学；生物效应；吸入毒性

科学通报，2015，60(8)：727-740.

13. 大气纳米颗粒物对人体健康效应的研究进展

Research advance on the health effects of nanoparticles in the air pollution in China

　　摘要：大气颗粒物中细颗粒物的健康危害已经得到证实，其中超细颗粒物（即纳米颗粒物）对人体健康的危害也逐渐得到研究者的关注。本文首先根据我国大气中存在的纳米颗粒物的特点，探讨了其来源和理化特性，然后重点总结了我国大气污染物中常见的纳米颗粒物对机体主要组织器官的负面生物效应和作用机制，最后提出了对大气污染物中纳米颗粒物的研究重点。

　　关键词：大气，纳米颗粒，健康状况，毒性

中华预防医学杂志，2015，49（9）：88-91.

14. 职业暴露可吸入性二氧化钛致心肺效应研究

A panel study for cardiopulmonary effects produced by occupational exposure to inhalable titanium dioxide

Abstract: OBJECTIVES: To investigate titanium dioxide TiO_2 exposure level in the finished product workshop, and its short-term cardiopulmonary effects, based on exposure assessment. METHODS: Seven workers were recruited into the panel. Personal TiO_2 exposure information, cardiopulmonary function, and the particle size distribution data were collected during working days. Linear mixed effect model was used to examine the association between TiO_2 exposure and cardiopulmonary function changes. RESULTS: The weight percentage of TiO_2 particles more than 10 μm, 1 to 10 μm, and less than 1 μm in the total dust was 14.5%, 69.5%, and 16%, respectively. Linear mixed effect model analysis showed that 1 mg/m increase in daily personal TiO_2 exposure was associated with the decline in maximum voluntary ventilation, peak expiratory flow, maximum mid-expiratory flow, and 75% of maximum expiratory flow. CONCLUSION: The study provided new evidence for health effects of occupational inhalable TiO_2 exposure, which suggests setting up new occupational exposure standards for fine TiO_2.

J. Occup. Environ. Med., 2012, 54(11):1389-1394.

15. 车间二氧化钛接触对职业人群氧化应激水平影响的定群研究

The effect of inhalable titanium dioxide on the oxidative stress among occupational population

　　摘要：目的：了解职业人群吸入性二氧化钛颗粒的接触水平，探讨其对工人机体氧化应激水平的影响。方法：应用定群设计的研究方法，通过问卷调查了解某二氧化钛生产车间成品岗位 7 名工人的一般信息及职业接触史，观察前后分别采集工人外周静脉血 10 mL，同时，连续 29 d 每日班前班后 30 min 内各采集尿样 30 mL（共 60 mL），并测定工人每日二氧化钛接触量及车间环境温、湿度。乳胶免疫比浊法测定个体外周血清超敏 C 反应蛋白（high-sensitivity C-reactive protein，hs-CRP）水平，酶联免疫吸附法（ELISA）测定尿 8-羟基脱氧鸟苷（8-hydroxy-deox-yguanosine，8-OHdG）水平。结果：个体每日接触可吸入性二氧化钛颗粒平均浓度为（1.194±1.015）mg/m^3；观察前后血样中 hs-CRP 水平分别为（1.13±1.08）、（1.33±1.01）mg/L，差异未见统计学意义（t＝−0.848，P＝0.425）；班前班后尿样中 8-OHdG 水平分别为（3.51±1.39）、（3.65±1.06）μmol/mol Cr。相关性分析显示，随着二氧化钛颗粒接触浓度的增加，8-OHdG 水平班前班后差异呈增大趋势（r＝0.192，t＝2.09，P＝0.039）。经班次、工龄、年龄、体质指数（BMI）等调整后，单污染物模型分析未发现二氧化钛浓度与班前班后 8-OHdG 水平差异存在统计学意义（β＝0.288，t＝1.940，P＝0.055）。结论：职业场所可吸入二氧化钛颗粒在所研究浓度范围，尚未发现工人机体 DNA 氧化应激水平发生明显变化。

　　关键词：钛；氧化合物；职业暴露；脱氧鸟苷；定群研究

中华预防医学杂志，2010，44（9）：775-779.

16. 电火花线切割加工车间空气中纳米颗粒污染以及潜在的健康危害
Airborne nanoparticle pollution in a wire electrical discharge machining workshop and potential health risks

Abstract: The environmental pollution associated with electrical discharge machining is not yet clearly understood. Airborne exposure to nanoscale and respirable particles were investigated with regard to the aerosol characteristics of a wire electrical discharge machining (WEDM) workshop. The total number concentration of the aerosol was multimodal, with the highest peak maxima during the working hours of 10:00 am and 3:00 pm. The majority of the released particles were smaller than d = 100 nm, with the maximum amount sized 40 nm. A large quantity of metallic elements, including Fe, Al and Cu, were found in the aerosol particulates coming from WEDM processing. Furthermore, the aerosol particles exhibited higher cellular toxicity and ROS producing ability in human alveolar epithelial cells (16HBE) when compared to the atmospheric background. Our results indicate substantial hazards arising from exposure to polluted atmosphere of a WEDM workshop. Effective exposure controls and protections are thus strongly recommended.

Keywords: aerosols; particle distribution; elemental concentration; risk assessment; toxicity

Aerosol Air Qual. Res., 2015, 15(1): 284-294.

17. 2013 年春节期间北京市大气颗粒物粒径范围表征及元素含量分析

Wide-range particle characterization and elemental concentration in Beijing aerosol during the 2013 spring festival

Abstract: The number and mass concentration, size distribution, and the concentration of 16 elements were studied in aerosol samples during the Spring Festival celebrations in 2013 in Beijing, China. Both the number and mass concentration increased sharply in a wide range from 10 nm to 10 μm during the firecrackers and fireworks activities. The prominent increase of the number concentration was in 50 nm-500 nm with a peak of $1.7 \times 10^5/cm^3$ at 150 nm, which is 8 times higher than that after 1.5 h. The highest mass concentration was in 320-560 nm, which is 4 times higher than the control. K, Mg, Sr, Ba and Pb increased sharply during the firework activities in PM10. Although the aerosol emission from firework activities is a short-term air quality degradation event, there may be a substantial hazard arising from the chemical composition of the emitted particles.

Keywords: Beijing; elemental concentration; firecrackers; fireworks; particle distribution; spring festival

Environ. Pollut., *2014*, *192*: *204-211*.

18. 碳纳米管吸附血液蛋白降低其细胞毒性
Binding of blood proteins to carbon nanotubes reduces cytotoxicity

Abstract: With the potential wide uses of nanoparticles such as carbon nanotubes in biomedical applications, and the growing concerns of nanotoxicity of these engineered nanoparticles, the importance of nanoparticle-protein interactions cannot be stressed enough. In this study, we use both experimental and theoretical approaches, including atomic force microscope images, fluorescence spectroscopy, CD, SDS-PAGE, and molecular dynamics simulations, to investigate the interactions of single-wall carbon nanotubes (SWCNTs) with human serum proteins, and find a competitive binding of these proteins with different adsorption capacity and packing modes. The π-π stacking interactions between SWCNTs and aromatic residues (Trp, Phe, Tyr) are found to play a critical role in determining their adsorption capacity. Additional cellular cytotoxicity assays, with human acute monocytic leukemia cell line and human umbilical vein endothelial cells, reveal that the competitive bindings of blood proteins on the SWCNT surface can greatly alter their cellular interaction pathways and result in much reduced cytotoxicity for these protein-coated SWCNTs, according to their respective adsorption capacity. These findings have shed light toward the design of safe carbon nanotube nanomaterials by comprehensive preconsideration of their interactions with human serum proteins.

Keywords: competitive adsorption; nanoparticle-protein corona; hydrophobic interactions; conformational flexibility

Proc. Natl. Acad. Sci. USA, 2011, 108 (41): 16968-16973.

19. 碳纳米管材料中金属杂质和管状结构对毒性的贡献
The contributions of metal impurities and tube structure to the toxicity of carbon nanotube materials

Abstract: Due to the existence of considerable quantities of metallic and carbonaceous impurities, the key factor and mechanism for the reported toxicity of carbon nanotubes (CNTs) are unclear. Here, we first quantify the contribution of metal residues and fiber structure to the toxicity of CNTs. Significant quantities of metal particles could be mobilized from CNTs into surrounding fluids, depending on the properties and constituents of the biological microenvironment, as well as the properties of metal particles. Furthermore, electron spin resonance measurements confirm that hydroxyl radicals can be generated by both CNTs containing metal impurities and acid-leachable metals from CNTs. Several biomolecules facilitate the generation of free radicals, which might be due to the participation of these biomolecules in redox cycling influenced by pH. Among several major metal residues, Fe has a critical role in generating hydroxyl radicals, reducing cell viability and promoting intracellular reactive oxidative species. Cell viability is highly dependent on the amount of metal residues and iron in particular, but not tube structure, while the negative effect of CNTs themselves on cell viability is very limited in a certain concentration range below 80 $\mu g\ mL^{-1}$. It is crucial to systematically understand how these exogenous and endogenous factors influence the toxicity of CNTs to avoid their undesirable toxicity.

Keywords: biological microenvironments; carbon nanotube; metal impurities; reactive oxygen species; toxicity

NPG Asia Mater., *2012*, *4*: *e32*.

20. 单壁碳纳米管导致自发高血压大鼠急性肺损伤与中度心血管效应

Acute pulmonary and moderate cardiovascular responses of spontaneously hypertensive rats after exposure to single-wall carbon nanotubes

Abstract：As a novel kind of nanomaterial with wide potential applications, the adverse effects of carbon nanotubes (CNTs) have recently received significant attention after respiratory exposure. In this study, single-wall carbon nanotubes (SWCNTs) containing different metal contents were intratracheally instilled into lungs of spontaneously hypertensive rats. Pulmonary and cardiovascular system alterations were evaluated at 24 and 72 h post-instillation. Biomarkers of inflammation, oxidative stress and cell damage in the bronchoalveolar lavage fluid (BALF) were increased significantly 24 h post-exposure of SWCNTs. The increased endothelin-1 levels in BALF and plasma and angiotensin I-converting enzyme in plasma suggested endothelial dysfunction in the pulmonary circulation and peripheral vascular thrombosis. These findings suggest that respiratory exposure to SWCNTs can induce acute pulmonary and cardiovascular responses and individuals with existing cardiovascular diseases are very susceptible to SWC-NTs exposure. The co-existence of metal residues in SWCNTs can aggravate the adverse effects.

Keywords：Intratracheal instillation; single-wall carbon nanotube; metal residues; cardiovascular effect; pulmonary toxicity

Nanotoxicology, 2012, 6(5)：526-542.

21. 多壁碳纳米管气管滴注自发高血压大鼠后的亚慢性毒性及心血管效应研究
Subchronic toxicity and cardiovascular responses in spontaneously hypertensive rats after exposure to multiwalled carbon nanotubes by intratracheal instillation

Abstract: The tremendous demand of the market for carbon nanotubes has led to their massive production that presents an increasing risk through occupational exposure. Lung deposition of carbon nanotubes is known to cause acute localized pulmonary adverse effects. However, systemic cardiovascular damages associated with acute pulmonary lesion have not been thoroughly addressed. Four kinds of multiwalled carbon nanotubes (MWCNTs) with different lengths and/or iron contents were used to explore the potential subchronic toxicological effects in spontaneously hypertensive (SH) rats and normotensive control Wistar-Kyoto (WKY) rats after intratracheal instillation. MWCNTs penetrated the lung blood-gas barrier and accumulated in the liver, kidneys, and spleen but not in the heart and aorta of SH rats. The pulmonary toxicity and cardiovascular effects were assessed at 7 and 30 days postexposure. Compared to the WKY rats, transient influences on blood pressure and up to 30 days persistent decrease in the heart rate of SH rats were found by electrocardiogram monitoring. The subchronic toxicity, especially the sustained inflammation of the pulmonary and cardiovascular system, was revealed at days 7 and 30 in both SH and WKY rat models. Histopathological results showed obvious morphological lesions in abdominal arteries of SH rats 30 days after exposure. Our results suggest that more attention should be paid to the long-term toxic effects of MWCNTs, and particularly, occupationally exposed workers with preexisting cardiovascular diseases should be monitored more thoroughly.

Chem. Res. Toxicol., 2015, 28(3):440-450.

22. 多壁碳纳米管通过激活 TGF-β/Smad 信号通路直接促进成纤维细胞向肌成纤维细胞转化和上皮间质转化

Multiwall carbon nanotubes directly promote fibroblast-myofibroblast and epithelial-mesenchymal transitions through the activation of the TGF-β/Smad signaling pathway

Abstract: A number of studies have demonstrated that MWCNTs induce granuloma formation and fibrotic responses in vivo, and it has been recently reported that MWCNT-induced macrophage activation and subsequent TGF-β secretion contribute to pulmonary fibrotic responses. However, their direct effects against alveolar type-II epithelial cells and fibroblasts and the corresponding underlying mechanisms remain largely unaddressed. Here, MWCNTs are reported to be able to directly promote fibroblast-to-myofibroblast conversion and the epithelial-mesenchymal transition (EMT) through the activation of the TGF-β/Smad signaling pathway. Both of the cell transitions may play important roles in MWCNT-induced pulmonary fibrosis. Firstly, in-vivo and in-vitro data show that long MWCNTs can directly interact with fibroblasts and epithelial cells, and some of them may be uptaken into fibroblasts and epithelial cells by endocytosis. Secondly, long MWCNTs can directly activate fibroblasts and increase both the basal and TGF-β1-induced expression of the fibroblast-specific protein-1, α-smooth muscle actin, and collagen III. Finally, MWCNTs can induce the EMT through the activation of TGF-β/Smad2 signaling in alveolar type-II epithelial cells, from which some fibroblasts involved in pulmonary fibrosis are thought to originate. These observations suggest that the activation of the TGF-β/Smad2 signaling plays a critical role in the process of the fibroblast-to-myofibroblast transition and the EMT induced by MWCNTs.

Keywords: MWCNTs; carbon nanotubes; cytotoxicity; materials biosafety; pulmonary fibrosis

Small, *2015*, *11*(4): 446-455.

23. 多壁碳纳米管通过 TGF-β/Smad 信号通路介导巨噬细胞活化和促进肺纤维化

Multiwall carbon nanotubes mediate macrophage activation and promote pulmonary fibrosis through TGF-β/Smad signaling pathway

Abstract: Multiwall carbon nanotubes (MWCNTs) have been widely used in many disciplines due to their unique physical and chemical properties, but have also raised great concerns about their possible negative health impacts, especially through occupational exposure. Although recent studies have demonstrated that MWCNTs induce granuloma formation and/or fibrotic responses in the lungs of rats or mice, their cellular and molecular mechanisms remain largely unaddressed. Here, it is reported that the TGF-β/Smad signaling pathway can be activated by MWCNTs and play a critical role in MWCNT-induced pulmonary fibrosis. Firstly, in vivo data show that spontaneously hypertensive (SH) rats administered long MWCNTs (20～50 μm) but not short MWCNTs (0.5～2 μm) exhibit increased fibroblast proliferation, collagen deposition and granuloma formation in lung tissue. Secondly, the in vivo experiments also indicate that only long MWCNTs can significantly activate macrophages and increase the production of transforming growth factor (TGF)-β1, which induces the phosphorylation of Smad2 and then the expression of collagen I/III and extracellular matrix (ECM) protease inhibitors in lung tissues. Finally, the present in vitro studies further demonstrate that the TGF-β/Smad signaling pathway is indeed necessary for the expression of collagen III in fibroblast cells. Together, these data demonstrate that MWCNTs stimulate pulmonary fibrotic responses such as fibroblast proliferation and collagen deposition in a TGF-β/Smad-dependent manner. These observations also suggest that tube length acts as an important factor in MWCNT-induced macrophage activation and subsequent TGF-β1 secretion. These in vivo and in vitro studies further highlight the potential adverse health effects that may occur following MWCNT exposure and provide a better understanding of the cellular and molecular mechanisms by which MWCNTs induce pulmonary fibrotic reactions.

Keywords: TGF-β/Smad signaling; collagen deposition; multiwall CNTs; pulmonary fibrosis

Small, 2013, 9(22): 3799-3811.

24. 多壁碳纳米管通过 TGF-β/Smad 信号通路实现上皮-间质转化诱导肺纤维化
Epithelial-mesenchymal transition involved in pulmonary fibrosis induced by multi-walled carbon nanotubes via TGF-beta/Smad signaling pathway

Abstract：Multi-walled carbon nanotubes (MWCNT) are a typical nanomaterial with a wide spectrum of commercial applications. Inhalation exposure to MWCNT has been linked with lung fibrosis and mesothelioma-like lesions commonly seen with asbestos. In this study, we examined the pulmonary fibrosis response to different length of MWCNT including short MWCNT (S-MWCNT, length=350～700nm) and long MWCNT (L-MWCNT, length=5～15 μm) and investigated whether the epithelial-mesenchymal transition (EMT) occurred during MWCNT-induced pulmonary fibrosis. C57Bl/6J male mice were intratracheally instilled with S-MWCNT or L-WCNT by a single dose of 60 μg per mouse, and the progress of pulmonary fibrosis was evaluated at 7, 28 and 56 days postexposure. The in vivo data showed that only L-MWCNT increased collagen deposition and pulmonary fibrosis significantly, and approximately 20% of pro-surfactant protein-C positive epithelial cells transdifferentiated to fibroblasts at 56 days, suggesting the occurrence of EMT. In order to understand the mechanism, we used human pulmonary epithelial cell line A549 to investigate the role of TGF-β/p-Smad2 signaling pathway in EMT. Our results showed that L-MWCNT downregulated E-cadherin and upregulated α-smooth muscle actin (α-SMA) protein expression in A549 cells. Taken together, both in vivo and in vitro study demonstrated that respiratory exposure to MWCNT induced length dependent pulmonary fibrosis and epithelial-derived fibroblasts via TGF-β/Smad pathway.

Keywords：Epithelial-mesenchymal transition; MWCNT; Pulmonary fibrosis; Smad; TGF-β

Toxicol. Lett., 2014, 226(2):150-162.

25. 多壁碳纳米管通过线粒体途径和吞噬受体诱导细胞凋亡
Multi-walled carbon nanotubes induce apoptosis *via* mitochondrial pathway and scavenger receptor

Abstract： We have demonstrated previously that the acid-treated multi-walled carbon nanotubes (aci-MWCNTs) and taurine functionalized MWCNTs (tau-MWCNTs) induced differential pulmonary toxicity in mice after instillation exposure. In order to compare differences of cytotoxicity between the aci-and tau-MWCNTs, RAW 264. 7 cells (a murine macrophage cell line) were chosen to be exposed to the aci-and tau-MWCNTs at concentrations of 0, 5, 20, 40, and 80 µg/ml for 12 or 24h respectively. The results showed that although the aci-and tau-MWCNTs induced only mild decrease in cell viability to RAW 264. 7 cells, the two types of MWCNTs elicited significant increase in apoptosis and decreased ability in cellular phagocytosis. Moreover, by using the specific inhibitors, we found that the scavenger receptors (SR) and caspase-9 were actively involved in the apoptosis induced by the aci-and tau-MWCNTs. The taurine functionalized MWCNTs (tau-MWCNTs) showed less cytotoxicity and apoptotic effect to RAW 264. 7 cells than those of aci-MWCNTs. Taken together, the results indicated the important role of scavenger receptors and mitochondria in the apoptosis induced by MWCNTs.

Keywords： Multi-walled carbon nanotubes (MWCNTs); RAW 264. 7 cells; apoptosis; scavenger receptors; mitochondria

Toxicol. in vitro, 2012, 26(6): 799-806.

26. 短多壁碳纳米管通过上调神经营养因子信号通路促进 PC12 神经细胞分化

Short multiwall carbon nanotubes promote neuronal differentiation of PC12 cells *via* up-regulation of the neurotrophin signaling pathway

Abstract：Numerous unique properties of carbon nanotubes make them attractive for applications in neurobiology such as drug delivery, tissue regeneration, and as scaffolds for neuronal growth. In this study, the critical roles of the length of multiwall carbon nanotubes (MWCNTs) on a neuronal-like model cell line PC12 cells are investigated. Incubation of PC12 cells with carboxylated MWCNTs did not significantly affect cellular morphology and viability at lower concentrations. Short MWCNTs show higher cellular uptake and more obvious removal compared to longer ones, which can result in higher ability to promote PC12 cell differentiation. Pre-incubation of short MWCNTs can up-regulate the expression of neurotrophin signaling pathway-associated TrkA/p75 receptors and Pincher/Gap43/TH proteins, which might be the underlying mechanism for the improved differentiation in PC12 cells. The current results provide insight for future applications of MWCNTs in neuron drug delivery and neurodegenerative disease treatment.

Keywords：carbon nanotubes; neuronal differentiation; PC12; growth factors; signaling pathways

Small, *2013*, *9(9-10)*：*1786-1798*.

27. 高铁杂质的多壁碳纳米管对 PC12 细胞活性和神经细胞分化的抑制作用

Inhibitory effects of multiwall carbon nanotubes with high iron impurity on viability and neuronal differentiation in cultured PC12 cells

Abstract：The increasing use of carbon nanotubes（CNTs）in biomedical applications has garnered a great concern on their potential negative effects to human health. CNTs have been reported to potentially disrupt normal neuronal function and they were speculated to accumulate and cause brain damage, although a lot of distinct and exceptional properties and potential wide applications have been associated with this material in neurobiology. Fe impurities strapped inside the CNTs may be partially responsible for neurotoxicity generation. In the present study, we selected rat pheochromocytoma（PC12）cells to investigate and compare the effects of two kinds of multiwall carbon nanotubes（MWCNTs）with different concentrations of Fe impurities which usually come from the massive production of CNTs by chemical vapor deposition. Exposure to Fe-high MWCNTs can reduce cell viability and increase cytoskeletal disruption of undifferentiated PC12 cells, diminish the ability to form mature neurites, and then adversely influence the neuronal dopaminergic phenotype in NGF-treated PC-12 cells. The present results highlight the critical role of iron residue in the adverse response to MWCNTs exposure in neural cells. These findings provide useful information for understanding the toxicity and safe application of carbon nanotubes.

Keywords：Differentiation；metal impurities；multiwall carbon nanotubes；neuron；neurotoxicity；pc12 cells

Toxicology, 2013, 313(1)：49-58.

28. 碳纳米材料的细胞毒性：单壁纳米管，多壁纳米管和富勒烯
Cytotoxicity of carbon nanomaterials: Single-wall nanotube, multi-wall nanotube, and fullerene

Abstract: A cytotoxicity test protocol for single-wall nanotubes (SWNTs), multi-wall nanotubes (with diameters ranging from 10 to 20 nm, MWNT10), and fullerene (C60) was tested. Profound cytotoxicity of SWNTs was observed in alveolar macrophage (AM) after a 6-h exposure *in vitro*. The cytotoxicity increases by as high as approximately 35% when the dosage of SWNTs was increased by 11.30 microg/cm^2. No significant toxicity was observed for C60 up to a dose of 226.00 microg/cm^2. The cytotoxicity apparently follows a sequence order on a mass basis: SWNTs>MWNT10>quartz>C60. SWNTs significantly impaired phagocytosis of AM at the low dose of 0.38 microg/cm^2, whereas MWNT10 and C60 induced injury only at the high dose of 3.06 microg/cm^2. The macrophages exposed to SWNTs or MWNT10 of 3.06 microg/cm^2 showed characteristic features of necrosis and degeneration. A sign of apoptotic cell death likely existed. Carbon nanomaterials with different geometric structures exhibit quite different cytotoxicity and bioactivity *in vitro*, although they may not be accurately reflected in the comparative toxicity *in vivo*.

Environ. Sci. Technol., 2005, 39(5): 1378-1383.

29. 碳纳米管对人体肠道细菌的广谱抗菌活性
Broad-spectrum antibacterial activity of carbon nanotubes to human gut bacteria

Abstract：Carbon nanotubes (CNTs) hold promise in manufacturing, environmental, and biomedical applications, as well as food and agricultural industries. Previous observations have shown that CNTs have antimicrobial activity; however, the impact of CNTs to human gut microbes has not been investigated. Here, the antibacterial activity of CNTs against the microbes commonly encountered in the human digestion system—*L. acidophilus*, *B. adolescentis*, *E. coli*, *E. faecalis*, and *S. aureus*-are evaluated. The bacteria studied include pathogenic and non-pathogenic, gram-positive and negative, and both sphere and rod strains. In this study, CNTs, including single-walled CNTs (SWCNTs, 1~3 μm), short and long multi-walled CNTs (s-MWCNTs: 0.5~2 μm; l-MWCNTs: >50 μm), and functionalized multi-walled CNTs (hydroxyl-and carboxyl-modification, 0.5~2 μm), all have broad-spectrum antibacterial effects. Notably, CNTs may selectively lyse the walls and membranes of human gut microbes, depending on not only the length and surface functional groups of CNTs, but also the shapes of the bacteria. The mechanism of antibacterial activity is associated with their diameter-dependent piercing and length-dependent wrapping on the lysis of microbial walls and membranes, inducing release of intracellular components DNA and RNA and allowing a loss of bacterial membrane potential, demonstrating complete destruction of bacteria. Thin and rigid SWCNT show more effective wall/membrane piercing on spherical bacteria than MWCNTs. Long MWCNT may wrap around gut bacteria, increasing the area making contact with the bacterial wall. This work suggests that CNTs may be broad-spectrum and efficient antibacterial agents in the gut, and selective application of CNTs could reduce the potential hazard to probiotic bacteria.

Keywords：antibacterials; carbon nanotubes; gut bacteria; membrane lysis

Small，2013，9(16)：2735-2746.

30. 体内多壁碳纳米管的转移和毒性受 microRNAs 调控
In vivo translocation and toxicity of multi-walled carbon nanotubes are regulated by microRNAs

Abstract: We employed an *in vivo* Caenorhabditis elegans assay system to perform SOLiD sequencing analysis to identify the possible microRNA (miRNA) targets of multi-walled carbon nanotubes (MWCNTs). Bioinformatics analysis on targeted genes for the identified dysregulated miRNAs in MWCNT exposed nematodes demonstrates their involvement in many aspects of biological processes. We used loss-of-function mutants for the identified dysregulated miRNAs to perform toxicity assessment by evaluating functions of primary and secondary targeted organs, and found the miRNA mutants with susceptible or resistant property towards MWCNT toxicity. Both the physiological state of the intestine and defecation behavior were involved in the control of the susceptible or resistant property occurrence for specific miRNA mutants towards MWCNT toxicity. This work provides the molecular basis at the miRNA level for future chemical design to reduce the nanotoxicity of MWCNTs and further elucidation of the related toxicological mechanism.

Nanoscale, 2014, 6(8): 4275-4284.

31. 多羟基金属富勒醇通过 TLRs/MyD88/NF-κB 和 NLRP3 炎症小体激活来刺激巨噬细胞分泌 IL-1β 细胞因子

Polyhydroxylated metallofullerenols stimulate IL-1β secretion of macrophage through TLRs/MyD88/NF-κB pathway and NLRP3 inflammasome activation

Abstract: Polyhydroxylated fullerenols especially gadolinium endohedral metallofullerenols $(Gd@C_{82}(OH)_{22})$ are shown as a promising agent for antitumor chemotherapeutics and good immunoregulatory effects with low toxicity. However, their underlying mechanism remains largely unclear. We found for the first time the persistent uptake and subcellular distribution of metallofullerenols in macrophages by taking advantages of synchrotron-based scanning transmission X-ray microscopy (STXM) with high spatial resolution of 30 nm. $Gd@C_{82}(OH)_{22}$ can significantly activate primary mouse macrophages to produce pro-inflammatory cytokines like IL-1β. Knockdown by small interfering RNA (siRNA) shows that it is NLRP3 inflammasomes but not NLRC4 participate in fullerenol-induced IL-1β production. Potassium efflux, activation of P2X7 receptor and intracellular reactive oxygen speciesare also important factors required for fullerenols-induced IL-1β release. Stronger NF-κB signal triggered by $Gd@C_{82}(OH)_{22}$ is in agreement with higher pro-IL-1β expression than $C_{60}(OH)_{22}$. Interestingly, TLR4/MyD88 pathway but not TLR2 mediates IL-1β secretion in $Gd@C_{82}(OH)_{22}$ exposure confirmed by macrophages from MyD88-/-/TLR4-/-/TLR2-/-knockout mice, which is different from $C_{60}(OH)_{22}$. Our work demonstrated that fullerenols can greatly activate macrophage and promote IL-1β production via both TLRs/MyD88/NF-κB pathway and NLRP3 inflammasome activation, while $Gd@C_{82}(OH)_{22}$ had stronger ability $C_{60}(OH)_{22}$ due to the different electron affinity on the surface of carbon cage induced by the encaged gadolinium ion.

Small, 2014, 10(12): 2362-2372.

32. 通过化学修饰银颗粒的表面进而影响其单次急性血液注射后的毒性和生物分布
Demonstrating approaches to chemically modify the surface of Ag nanoparticles in order to influence their cytotoxicity and biodistribution after single dose acute intravenous administration

Abstract: With the advance in material science and the need to diversify market applications, silver nanoparticles (AgNPs) are modified by different surface coatings. However, how these surface modifications influence the effects of AgNPs on human health is still largely unknown. We have evaluated the uptake, toxicity and pharmacokinetics of AgNPs coated with citrate, polyethylene glycol, polyvinyl pyrolidone and branched polyethyleneimine (Citrate AgNPs, PEG AgNPs, PVP AgNPs and BPEI AgNPs, respectively). Our results demonstrated that the toxicity of AgNPs depends on the intracellular localization that was highly dependent on the surface charge. BPEI AgNPs (Zeta potential $+46.5$ mV) induced the highest cytotoxicity and DNA fragmentation in Hepa1c1c7. In addition, it showed the highest damage to the nucleus of liver cells in the exposed mice, which is associated with a high accumulation in liver tissues. The PEG AgNPs (Zeta potential-16.2 mV) showed the cytotoxicity, a long blood circulation, as well as bioaccumulation in spleen (34.33 mg/g), which suggest better biocompatibility compared to the other chemically modified AgNPs. Moreover, the adsorption ability with bovine serum albumin revealed that the PEG surface of AgNPs has an optimal biological inertia and can effectively resist opsonization or non-specific binding to protein in mice. The overall results indicated that the biodistribution of AgNPs was significantly dependent on surface chemistry: BPEI AgNPs>Citrate AgNPs=PVP AgNPs>PEG AgNPs. This toxicological data could be useful in supporting the development of safe AgNPs for consumer products and drug delivery applications.

Nanotoxicology, *DOI*: *10.3109/17435390.2015.1024295*

33. 同步辐射相关分析揭示纳米银毒性的化学变化机理

Use of synchrotron radiation-analytical techniques to reveal chemical origin of silver-nanoparticle cytotoxicity

Abstract: To predict potential medical value or toxicity of nanoparticles (NPs), it is necessary to understand the chemical transformation during intracellular processes of NPs. However, it is a grand challenge to capture a high-resolution image of metallic NPs in a single cell and the chemical information on intracellular NPs. Here, by integrating synchrotron radiation-beam transmission X-ray microscopy (SR-TXM) and SR-X-ray absorption near edge structure (SR-XANES) spectroscopy, we successfully capture the 3D distribution of silver NPs (AgNPs) inside a single human monocyte (THP-1), associated with the chemical transformation of silver. The results reveal that the cytotoxicity of AgNPs is largely due to the chemical transformation of particulate silver from elemental silver (Ag(0))n, to Ag(+) ions and Ag-O-, then Ag-S-species. These results provide direct evidence in the long-lasting debate on whether the nanoscale or the ionic form dominates the cytotoxicity of silver nanoparticles. Further, the present approach provides an integrated strategy capable of exploring the chemical origins of cytotoxicity in metallic nanoparticles.

Keywords: AgNPs; chemical origin; chemical transformation; dynamic processes of intracellular nanoparticles; nano-CT; nanotoxicity

ACS Nano, 2015, 9(6): 6532-6547.

34. 纳米银在细胞与小鼠模型中激活内质网应激信号通路及相关毒理学评价应用
Silver nanoparticles activate endoplasmic reticulum stress signaling pathway in cell and mouse models: The role in toxicity evaluation

Abstract: Silver nanoparticles (AgNPs) attract considerable public attention both for their antimicrobial properties and their potential adverse effects. In the present study, endoplasmic reticulum (ER) stress was used as a sensitive and early biomarker to evaluate the toxic potential of AgNPs in three different human cell lines in vitro and in vivo in mice. In 16HBE cells, the activation of ER stress signaling pathway was observed by upregulated expression including xbp-1s, chop/DDIT3, TRIB3, ADM2, BIP, Caspase-12, ASNS and HERP at either the mRNA and/or protein levels. However, these changes were not observed in HUVECs or HepG2 cells. Furthermore, mice experiments showed that different tissues had various sensitivities to AgNPs following intratracheal instillation exposure. The lung, liver and kidney showed significant ER stress responses, however, only the lung and kidney exhibited apoptosis by TUNEL assay. The artery and tracheal tissues had lower ER stress and apoptosis after exposure. The lowest observable effect concentrations (LOEC) were proposed based on evaluation of AgNP induced ER stress response in cell and mouse models. In summary, preliminary evaluation of AgNP toxicity by monitoring the ER stress signaling pathway provides new insights toward the understanding the biological impacts of AgNPs. The adverse effects of exposure to AgNPs may be avoided by rational use within the safe dose.

Keywords: Apoptosis; cytotoxicity; intratracheal instillation; signaling pathway; silver

Biomaterials, 2015, 61: 307-315.

35. 纳米银细胞毒性机理：CHO-K1 细胞持续内吞并在胞内快速溶解

Fast intracellular dissolution and persistent cellular uptake of silver nanoparticles in CHO-K1 cells: Implication for cytotoxicity

Abstract: Toxicity of silver nanoparticles (Ag NPs) has been reported both in vitro and in vivo. However, the intracellular stability and chemical state of Ag NPs are still not very well studied. In this work, we systematically investigated the cellular uptake pathways, intracellular dissolution and chemical species, and cytotoxicity of Ag NPs (15.9±7.6 nm) in Chinese hamster ovary cell subclone K1 cells, a cell line recommended by the OECD for genotoxicity studies. Quantification of intracellular nanoparticle uptake and ion release was performed through inductively coupled plasma mass spectrometry. X-ray absorption near-edge structure (XANES) was employed to assess the chemical state of intracellular silver. The toxic potential of Ag NPs and Ag(+) was evaluated by cell viability, reactive oxygen species (ROS) production and live-dead cell staining. The results suggest that cellular uptake of Ag NPs involves lipid-raft-mediated endocytosis and energy-independent diffusion. The degradation study shows that Ag NPs taken up into cells dissolved quickly and XANES results directly indicated that the internalized Ag was oxidized to Ag-O-species and then stabilized in silver-sulfur (Ag-S-) bonds within the cells. Subsequent cytotoxicity studies show that Ag NPs decrease cell viability and increase ROS production. Pre-incubation with N-acetyl-L-cysteine, an efficient antioxidant and Ag(+) chelator, diminished the cytotoxicity caused by Ag NPs or Ag(+) exposure. Our study suggests that the cytotoxicity mechanism of Ag NPs is related to the intracellular release of silver ions, followed by their binding to SH-groups, presumably coming from amino acids or proteins, and affecting protein functions and the antioxidant defense system of cells.

Keywords: Degradation; N-acetyl-l-cysteine; XANES; reactive oxygen species; silver nanoparticles; uptake pathway

Nanotoxicology, 2015, 9(2): 181-189.

36. 同步辐射技术揭示金纳米棒与蛋白冠的复合结构，理解细胞膜损伤降低的机理
Revealing the binding structure of the protein corona on gold nanorods using synchrotron radiation-based techniques: Understanding the reduced damage in cell membranes

Abstract: Regarding the importance of the biological effects of nanomaterials, there is still limited knowledge about the binding structure and stability of the protein corona on nanomaterials and the subsequent impacts. Here we designed a hard serum albumin protein corona (BSA) on CTAB-coated gold nanorods (AuNRs) and captured the structure of protein adsorption using synchrotron radiation X-ray absorption spectroscopy, microbeam X-ray fluorescent spectroscopy, and circular dichroism in combination with molecular dynamics simulations. The protein adsorption is attributed to at least 12 Au-S bonds and the stable corona reduced the cytotoxicity of CTAB/AuNRs. These combined strategies using physical, chemical, and biological approaches will improve our understanding of the protective effects of protein coronas against the toxicity of nanomaterials. These findings have shed light on a new strategy for studying interactions between proteins and nanomaterials, and this information will help further guide the rational design of nanomaterials for safe and effective biomedical applications.

J. Am. Chem. Soc. , 2013 , 135(46): 17359-17368.

37. 金纳米棒表面化学：细胞膜损伤和细胞毒性的根源
Surface chemistry of gold nanorods: origin of cell membrane damage and cytotoxicity

Abstract: We investigated how surface chemistry influences the interaction between gold nanorods (AuNRs) and cell membranes and the subsequent cytotoxicity arising from them in a serum-free cell culture system. Our results showed that the AuNRs coated with cetyl trimethylammonium bromide (CTAB) molecules can generate defects in the cell membrane and induce cell death, mainly due to the unique bilayer structure of CTAB molecules on the surface of the rods rather than their charge. Compared to CTAB-capped nanorods, positively charged polyelectrolyte-coated, i. e. poly(diallyldimethyl ammonium chloride) (PDDAC), AuNRs show improved biocompatibility towards cells. Thus, the present results indicate that the nature of surface molecules, especially their packing structures on the surface of AuNRs rather than surface charge, play a more crucial role in determining cytotoxicity. These findings about interfacial interactions could also explain the effects of internalized AuNRs on the structures or functions of organelles. This study will help understanding of the toxic nature of AuNRs and guide rational design of the surface chemistry of AuNRs for good biocompatibility in pharmaceutical therapy.

Nanoscale, 2013, 5(18): 8384-8391.

38. 金纳米棒的表面化学和长径比介导细胞摄取
Surface chemistry and aspect ratio mediated cellular uptake of Au nanorods

Abstract: Gold nanorods (Au NRs) have been recognized as promising materials for biomedical applications, like sensing, imaging, gene and drug delivery and therapy, but their toxicological issues are still controversial, especially for the Au NRs synthesized with seed-mediated method. In this study, we investigated the influence of aspect ratio and surface coating on their toxicity and cellular uptake. The cellular uptake is highly dependent on the aspect ratio and surface coating. However, the surface chemistry has the dominant roles since PDDAC-coated Au NRs exhibit a much greater ability to be internalized by the cells. The present data demonstrated shape-independent but coating-dependent cytotoxicity. Both the CTAB molecules left in the suspended solution and on the surface of Au NRs were identified as the actual cause of cytotoxicity. CTAB can enter cells with or without Au NRs, damage mitochondria, and then induce apoptosis. The effects of surface coating upon toxicity and cellular uptake were also examined using Au NRs with different coatings. When Au NRs were added into the medium, the proteins were quickly adsorbed onto the Au NRs that made the surface negatively charged. The surface charge may not directly affect the cellular uptake. We further demonstrated that the amount of serum proteins, especially for BSA, adsorbed on the Au NRs had a positive correlation with the capacity of Au NRs to enter cells. In addition, we have successfully revealed that the cationic PDDAC-coated Au NRs with an aspect ratio of 4 possess an ideal combination of both negligible toxicity and high cellular uptake efficiency, showing a great promise as photothermal therapeutic agents.

Keywords: Gold; nanoparticles; nanorods; cytotoxicity; aspect ratio; surface modification

Biomaterials, 2010, 31(30): 7606-7619.

39. 细胞对纳米材料的反应:胞外体作为肺外信号传送者起始纳米颗粒诱导的全身免疫激活

Cellular responses to nanomaterials: exosomes as extrapulmonary signaling conveyors for nanoparticle-induced systemic immune activation

Abstract: Evaluation of systemic biosafety of nanomaterials urgently demands a comprehensive understanding of the mechanisms of the undesirable interference and systemic signaling that arises between man-made nanomaterials and biological systems. It is shown that exosomes may act as signal conveyors for nanoparticle-induced systemic immune responses. Exosomes are extracellularly secreted membrane vesicles which act as Trojan horses for the dissemination and intercellular communication of natural nanosized particles (like viruses). Upon exposure to magnetic iron oxide nanoparticles (MIONs), it is possible to dose-dependently generate a significant number of exosomes in the alveolar region of BALB/c mice. These exosomes are quickly eliminated from alveoli into systemic circulation and largely transfer their signals to the immune system. Maturation of dendritic cells and activation of splenic T cells are significantly induced by these exosomes. Furthermore, exosome-induced T-cell activation is more efficient toward sensitized T cells and in ovalbumin (OVA)-sensitized mice than in the unsensitized counterparts. Activation of systemic T cells reveals a T helper 1 polarization and aggravated inflammation, which poses potential hazards to the deterioration of allergic diseases in OVA-sensitized mice. The studies suggest that exosomes may act as conveyors for extrapulmonary signal transduction in nanoparticle-induced immune systemic responses, which are the key in vivo processes of manufactured nanoparticles executing either biomedical functions or toxic responses.

Keywords: exosomes; iron; nanoparticles; signal transduction; systemic immune activation

Small, 2012, 8(3):404-412.

40. 纳米颗粒诱导形成的分泌囊泡靶向抗原递呈细胞启动 Th1 型免疫活化
Nanoparticle-induced exosomes target antigen-presenting cells to initiate Th1-type immune activation

Abstract：The mechanisms associated with the induction of systemic immune responses by nanoparticles are not fully understood, but their elucidation is critical to address safety issues associated with the broader medical application of nanotechnology. In this study, a key role of nanoparticle-induced exosomes (extracellularly secreted membrane vesicles) as signaling mediators in the induction of T helper cell type 1 (Th1) immune activation is demonstrated. In vivo exposure to magnetic iron oxide nanoparticles (MIONs) results in significant exosome generation in the alveolar region of Balb/c mice. These act as a source of nanoparticle-induced, membrane-bound antigen/signaling cargo, which transfer their components to antigen-presenting cells (APCs) in the reticuloendothelial system. Through exosome-initiated signals, immature dendritic cells (iDCs) undergo maturation and differentiation to the DC1 subtype, while macrophages go through classical activation and differentiation to the M1 subtype. Simultaneously, iDCs and macrophages release various Th1 cytokines (including interleukin-12 and tumor necrosis factor α) driving T-cell activation and differentiation. Activated APCs (especially DC1 and M1 subtypes) consequently prime T-cell differentiation towards a Th1 subtype, thereby resulting in an orchestrated Th1-type immune response. Th1-polarized immune activation is associated with delayed-type hypersensitivity, which might underlie the long-term inflammatory effects frequently associated with nanoparticle exposure. These studies suggest that nanoparticle-induced exosomes provoke the immune activation and inflammatory responses that can accompany nanoparticle exposure.

Keywords：cells; exosomes; immune response; magnetic materials; nanoparticles

Small, 2012, 8(18): 2841-2848.

41. 纳米氧化铁颗粒暴露引起的内皮细胞功能障碍和炎症是早期动脉粥样硬化的危险因素

Endothelial dysfunction and inflammation induced by iron oxide nanoparticle exposure: Risk factors for early atherosclerosis

Abstract: More recently, the correlation between exposure to nanoparticles and cardiovascular diseases is of particular concern in nanotoxicology related fields. Nanoparticle-triggered endothelial dysfunction is hypothesized to be a dominant mechanism in the development of the diseases. To test this hypothesis, iron oxide nanoparticles (Fe_2O_3 and Fe_3O_4), as two widely used nanomaterials and the main metallic components in particulate matter, were selected to assess their potential risks on human endothelial system. The direct effects of iron oxide nanoparticles on human aortic endothelial cells (HAECs) and the possible effects mediated by monocyte (U937 cells) phagocytosis and activation were investigated. In the study, HAECs and U937 cells were exposed to 2, 20, 100 μg/mL of 22-nm-Fe_2O_3 and 43-nm-Fe_3O_4 particles. Our results indicate that cytoplasmic vacuolation, mitochondrial swelling and cell death were induced in HAEC. A significant increase in nitric oxide (NO) production was induced which coincided with the elevation of nitric oxide synthase (NOS) activity in HAECs. Adhesion of monocytes to the HAECs was significantly enhanced as a consequence of the up-regulation of intracellular cell adhesion molecule-1 (ICAM-1) and interleukin-8 (IL-8) expression, all of which are considered as early steps of atherosclerosis. Phagocytosis and dissolution of nanoparticles by monocytes were found to simultaneously provoke oxidative stress and mediate severe endothelial toxicity. We conclude that intravascular iron oxide nanoparticles may induce endothelial system inflammation and dysfunction by three ways: (1) nanoparticles may escape from phagocytosis that interact directly with the endothelial monolayer; (2) nanoparticles are phagocytized by monocytes and then dissolved, thus impact the endothelial cells as free iron ions; or (3) nanoparticles are phagocytized by monocytes to provoke oxidative stress responses.

Keywords: Iron oxide nanoparticle; human aortic endothelial cells; atherosclerosis; endothelial dysfunction; human monocyte

Toxicol. Lett., 2011, 203(2): 162-171.

42. 纳米氧化铁颗粒暴露相关联的小胶质细胞活化，招募和吞噬现象
Microglial activation, recruitment and phagocytosis as linked phenomena in ferric oxide nanoparticle exposure.

Abstract: Microglia as the resident macrophage-like cells in the central nervous system (CNS) play a pivotal role in the innate immune responses of CNS. Understanding the reactions of microglia cells to nanoparticle exposure is important in the exploration of neurobiology of nanoparticles. Here we provide a systemic mapping of microglia and the corresponding pathological changes in olfactory-transport related brain areas of mice with Fe_2O_3-nanoparticle intranasal treatment. We showed that intranasal exposure of Fe_2O_3 nanoparticle could lead to pathological alteration in olfactory bulb, hippocampus and striatum, and caused microglial proliferation, activation and recruitment in these areas, especially in olfactory bulb. Further experiments with BV2 microglial cells showed the exposure to Fe_2O_3 nanoparticles could induce cells proliferation, phagocytosis and generation of ROS and NO, but did not cause significant release of inflammatory factors, including IL-1β, IL-6 and TNF-α. Our results indicate that microglial activation may act as an alarm and defense system in the processes of the exogenous nanoparticles invading and storage in brain.

Keywords: Ferric oxide nanoparticles; neurotoxicity; microglial activation

Toxicol. Lett., *2011*, *205(1)*: *26-37.*

43. 利用秀丽线虫模式生物全面评估量子点的代谢和生理行为

Full assessment of fate and physiological behavior of quantum dots utilizing caenorhabditis elegans as a model organism

Abstract: We evaluated the in vivo fate and physiological behavior of quantum dots (QDs) in Caenorhabditis elegans by GFP transfection, fluorescent imaging, synchrotron radiation based elemental imaging, and speciation techniques. The in situ metabolism and degradation of QDs in the alimentary system and long-term toxicity on reproduction are fully assessed. This work highlights the utility of the *C. elegans* model as a multiflexible platform to allow noninvasively imaging and monitoring in vivo consequences of engineered nanomaterials.

Keywords: *C. Elegans*; quantum dots; biodistribution; chemical speciation; in vivo imaging; reproductive toxicity

Nano Lett, 2011, 11(8): 3174-3183.

44. 量子点表面包覆的谷胱甘肽手性特征影响其毒性
Chirality of glutathione surface coating affects the cytotoxicity of quantum dots

Abstract：Choose your poison：Chiral CdTe quantum dots（QDs）coated with L-or D-glutathione（GSH）stabilizers exhibit differences in cytotoxicity although they have identical composition and size. D-GSH-QDs are less cytotoxic than L-GSH-QDs. The ability of QDs to induce cell death is correlated with their ability to induce autophagy，which is chirality-dependent.

Keywords：autophagy；chirality；cytotoxicity；fluorescence；quantum dots

Angew. Chem. Int. Ed.，*2011*，*50*（*26*）：*5860-5864*.

45. 不同含 CD 量子点对细胞周期和细胞分裂的影响

The influence on cell cycle and cell division by various cadmium-containing quantum dots

Abstract：Quantum dots (QDs) have attracted great attention because of their favorable optical properties and have been widely applied in biomedical fields. However, in recent years, there have been an increasing number of reports about the cytotoxicity of QDs, especially cadmium-containing QDs, which may release cadmium ions to induce cytotoxicity. Importantly, the chemical composition and surface modifications of cadmium-based QDs determine the amount of Cd^{2+} released inside the cell. Thus, there is an urgent need for more systematic work to study the relationship between cytotoxicity and the surface properties of QDs. In this article, the cytotoxicity of seven cadmium-containing QDs with different constituent elements and surface chemistries are compared. The results show that the cytotoxicity of QDs is closely related to their constituent elements and surface properties：First, CdTe@ZnS core-shell QDs show much lower cytotoxicity than naked ones when they have similar surface modifications; second, the positively charged QDs are more toxic than the negatively charged ones. Moreover, both positively and negatively charged QDs without ZnS coatings lead to multipolar spindles, misaligned chromosomes, and G2/M checkpoint failures. Interestingly, although CdSe QDs with a PEG coating cause no apparent cytotoxicity in any of the cell lines studied, they can localize near the contractile ring during cytokinesis and then block contractile ring disassembly. The cellular effect of CdTe QDs comes not only from the release of cadmium ions but also the intracellular distribution of QD nanoparticles in cells and the associated nanoscale effects. It is also found that QD-caused cytokinesis failure is closely related to the decreased expression of Cyclin A and Cyclin B. Taken together, the above findings provide new insight into the dynamic fate of QDs during cell mitosis, and are important for understanding the intracellular effects of QDs on the mitotic spindle and chromosomes during cell division. Furthermore, this kind of cytotoxicity evaluation method should be applicable to studies of the biological effects and health impacts of other nanomaterials.

Small 2013，9(14)：2440-2451.

46. 氧化石墨烯应激毒性特征及相关机理

Unraveling stress-induced toxicity properties of graphene oxide and the underlying mechanism

Abstract：Graphene oxide shows stress-induced toxicity properties in vivo under different pathophysiological conditions. A dual-path chemical mechanism，involving the overproduction of hydroxyl radicals and the formation of oxidizing cytochrome c intermediates，is responsible for the toxicity properties.

Adv. Mater.，2012，24(39)：5391-5397.

47. 秀丽线虫评价 Gd@C$_{82}$(OH)$_{22}$纳米粒子的生物安全性
Biosafety assessment of Gd@C$_{82}$(OH)$_{22}$ nanoparticles on *Caenorhabditis elegans*

Abstract：Gd@C$_{82}$(OH)$_{22}$, a water-soluble endohedral metallofullerene derivative, has been proven to possess significant antineoplastic activity in mice. Toxicity studies of the nanoparticle have shown some evidence of low or non toxicity in mice and cell models. Here we employed *Caenorhabditis elegans* (*C. elegans*) as a model organism to further evaluate the short-and long-term toxicity of Gd@C$_{82}$(OH)$_{22}$ and possible behavior changes under normal and stress culture conditions. With treatment of Gd@C$_{82}$(OH)$_{22}$ at 0.01, 0.1, 1.0 and 10 μg ml (−1) within one generation (short-term), *C. elegans* showed no significant decrease in longevity or thermotolerance compared to the controls. Furthermore, when Gd@C$_{82}$(OH)$_{22}$ treatment was extended up to six generations (long-term), non-toxic effects to the nematodes were found. In addition, data from body length measurement, feeding rate and egg-laying assays with short-term treatment demonstrated that the nanoparticles have no significant impact on the individual growth, feeding behavior and reproductive ability, respectively. In summary, this work has shown that Gd@C$_{82}$(OH)$_{22}$ is tolerated well by worms and it has no apparent toxic effects on longevity, stress resistance, growth and behaviors that were observed in both adult and young worms. Our work lays the foundations for further developments of this anti-neoplastic agent for clinical applications.

Nanoscale, 2011, 3(6): 2636-2641.

48. 秀丽线虫评价富勒醇对衰老及应激反应的影响

Evaluation of the influence of fullerenol on aging and stress resistance using *Caenorhabditis elegans*

Abstract：Fullerene derivatives have attracted extensive attention in biomedical fields and polyhydroxyl fullerene (fullerenol), a water-soluble fullerene derivative, is demonstrated as a powerful antioxidant. To further assess their anti-aging and anti-stress potential, we employed *Caenorhabditis elegans* (*C. elegans*) as a model organism to evaluate the effects of fullerenol on the growth, development, behavior and anti-stress ability *in vivo*. The data show that fullerenol has no obviously toxic effect on nematodes and can delay *C. elegans* aging progress under normal condition. Further studies demonstrate that fullerenol attenuates endogenous levels of reactive oxygen species and provides protection to *C. elegans* under stress conditions by up-regulating stress-related genes in a DAF-16 depend manner and improving lifespan. In summary, our data suggest that fullerenol might be a safe and reasonable anti-aging candidate with great potential in vivo.

Keywords：Anti-aging; caenorhabditis elegans; daf-16; fullerenol; insulin/IGF-1 pathway; lifespan

Biomaterials，2015，42：78-86.

49. 纳米氧化锌诱导的内质网应激可作为纳米毒理学评价的早期生物标志物
Endoplasmic reticulum stress induced by zinc oxide nanoparticles is an earlier biomarker for nanotoxicological evaluation

Abstract：Zinc oxide nanoparticles (ZnO NPs) have been widely used in cosmetics and sunscreens, advanced textiles, self-charging and electronic devices; the potential for human exposure and the health impact at each stage of their manufacture and use are attracting great concerns. In addition to pulmonary damage, nanoparticle exposure is also strongly correlated with the increase in incidences of cardiovascular diseases; however, their toxic potential remains largely unclear. Herein, we investigated the cellular responses and endoplasmatic reticulum (ER) stress induced by ZnO NPs in human umbilical vein endothelial cells (HUVECs) in comparison with the Zn^{2+} ions and CeO_2 NPs. We found that the dissolved zinc ion was the most significant factor for cytotoxicity in HUVECs. More importantly, ZnO NPs at noncytotoxic concentration, but not CeO_2 NPs, can induce significant cellular ER stress response with higher expression of spliced xbp-1, chop, and caspase-12 at the mRNA level, and associated ER marker proteins including BiP, Chop, GADD34, p-PERK, p-eIF2α, and cleaved Caspase-12 at the protein levels. Moreover, ER stress was widely activated after treatment with ZnO NPs, while six of 84 marker genes significantly increased. ER stress response is a sensitive marker for checking the interruption of ER homeostasis by ZnO NPs. Furthermore, higher dosage of ZnO NPs (240 μM) quickly rendered ER stress response before inducing apoptosis. These results demonstrate that ZnO NPs activate ER stress-responsive pathway and the ER stress response might be used as an earlier and sensitive end point for nanotoxicological study.

Keywords：ZnO; ceria; nanoparticles; ER stress; signaling pathways; cytotoxicity; apoptosis

ACS Nano, *2014*, *8(3)*：*2562-2574*.

50. 生物医学成像揭示无机纳米材料毒性
Toxicity of inorganic nanomaterials in biomedical imaging

Abstract: Inorganic nanoparticles have shown promising potentials as novel biomedical imaging agents with high sensitivity, high spatial and temporal resolution. To translate the laboratory innovations into clinical applications, their potential toxicities are highly concerned and have to be evaluated comprehensively both *in vitro* and *in vivo* before their clinical applications. In this review, we first summarized the *in vivo* and *in vitro* toxicities of the representative inorganic nanoparticles used in biomedical imagings. Then we further discuss the origin of nanotoxicity of inorganic nanomaterials, including ROS generation and oxidative stress, chemical instability, chemical composition, the surface modification, dissolution of nanoparticles to release excess free ions of metals, metal redox state, and left-over chemicals from synthesis, etc. We intend to provide the readers a better understanding of the toxicology aspects of inorganic nanomaterials and knowledge for achieving optimized designs of safer inorganic nanomaterials for clinical applications.

Keywords: gold nanoparticles; inorganic materials; iron nanoparticles; medical imaging; nanomedicine; nanotoxicity; QDs; upconversion nanoparticles

Biotechnol. Adv., 2014, 32(4): 727-743.

51. 蛋白质和碳相关纳米颗粒之间的相互作用：从分子水平探索毒性的根源

Interactions between proteins and carbon-based nanoparticles: Exploring the origin of nanotoxicity at molecular level

Abstract: The widespread application of nanomaterials has spurred an interest in the study of interactions between nanoparticles and proteins due to the biosafety concerns of these nanomaterials. In this review, a summary is presented of some of the recent studies on this important subject, especially on the interactions of proteins with carbon nanotubes (CNTs) and metallofullerenols. Two potential molecular mechanisms have been proposed for CNTs' inhibition of protein functions. The driving forces of CNTs' adsorption onto proteins are found to be mainly hydrophobic interactions and the so-called π-π stacking between CNTs' carbon rings and proteins' aromatic residues. However, there is also recent evidence showing that endohedral metallofullerenol $Gd@C_{82}(OH)_{22}$ can be used to inhibit tumor growth, thus acting as a potential nanomedicine. These recent findings have provided a better understanding of nanotoxicity at the molecular level and also suggested therapeutic potential by using nanoparticles' cytotoxicity against cancer cells.

Keywords: nanotoxicology; protein-nanoparticle interactions; molecular simulations; carbon nanotubes

Small, 2013, 9(9-10): 1546-1556.

52. 口香糖中纳米二氧化钛添加剂的表征与初步毒性分析

Characterization and preliminary toxicity assay of nano-titanium dioxide additive in sugar-coated chewing gum

Abstract: Nanotechnology shows great potential for producing food with higher quality and better taste through including new additives, improving nutrient delivery, and using better packaging. However, lack of investigations on safety issues of nanofood has resulted in public fears. How to characterize engineered nanomaterials in food and assess the toxicity and health impact of nanofood remains a big challenge. Herein, a facile and highly reliable separation method of TiO_2 particles from food products (focusing on sugar-coated chewing gum) is reported, and the first comprehensive characterization study on food nanoparticles by multiple qualitative and quantitative methods is provided. The detailed information on nanoparticles in gum includes chemical composition, morphology, size distribution, crystalline phase, particle and mass concentration, surface charge, and aggregation state. Surprisingly, the results show that the number of food products containing nano-TiO_2 (<200 nm) is much larger than known, and consumers have already often been exposed to engineered nanoparticles in daily life. Over 93% of TiO_2 in gum is nano-TiO_2, and it is unexpectedly easy to come out and be swallowed by a person who chews gum. Preliminary cytotoxicity assays show that the gum nano-TiO_2 particles are relatively safe for gastrointestinal cells within 24 h even at a concentration of 200 μg mL^{-1}. This comprehensive study demonstrates accurate physicochemical property, exposure, and cytotoxicity information on engineered nanoparticles in food, which is a prerequisite for the successful safety assessment of nanofood products.

Keywords: characterization; cytotoxicity; food additives; nanoparticles; titanium dioxide

Small, *2013*, *9(9-10)*: *1765-1774*.

53. 金红石型二氧化钛颗粒在小鼠脑内滞留与形成的损伤取决于颗粒大小和表面包被

Rutile TiO₂ particles exert size and surface coating dependent retention and lesions on the murine brain

Abstract: The rising commercial use and large-scale production of engineered nanoparticles (NPs) may lead to unintended exposure to humans. The central nervous system (CNS) is a potential susceptible target of the inhaled NPs, but so far the amount of studies on this aspect is limited. Here, we focus on the potential neurological lesion in the brain induced by the intranasally instilled titanium dioxide (TiO₂) particles in rutile phase and of various sizes and surface coatings. Female mice were intranasally instilled with four different types of TiO₂ particles (i. e. two types of hydrophobic particles in micro-and nano-sized without coating and two types of water-soluble hydrophilic nano-sized particles with silica surface coating) every other day for 30 days. Inductively coupled plasma mass spectrometry (ICP-MS) were used to determine the titanium contents in the sub-brain regions. Then, the pathological examination of brain tissues and measurements of the monoamine neurotransmitter levels in the sub-brain regions were performed. We found significant up-regulation of Ti contents in the cerebral cortex and striatum after intranasal instillation of hydrophilic TiO₂ NPs. Moreover, TiO₂ NPs exposure, in particular the hydrophilic NPs, caused obvious morphological changes of neurons in the cerebral cortex and significant disturbance of the monoamine neurotransmitter levels in the sub-brain regions studied. Thus, our results indicate that the surface modification of the NPs plays an important role on their effects on the brain. In addition, the difference in neurotoxicity of the two types of hydrophilic NPs may be induced by the shape differences of the materials. The present results suggest that physicochemical properties like size, shape and surface modification of the nanomaterials should be considered when evaluating their neurological effects.

Keywords: TiO₂ nanoparticles; surface modification; shape; intranasal instillation; neurotransmitter secretion; nanomaterials; murine brain; toxicity

Toxicol. Lett. , 2011, 207(1): 73-81.

54. 氧化锌,二氧化钛,二氧化硅和氧化铝纳米颗粒诱导人胚肺成纤维细胞毒性作用

ZnO, TiO$_2$, SiO$_2$, and Al$_2$O$_3$ nanoparticles-induced toxic effects on human fetal lung fibroblasts

Abstract: OBJECTIVE: This study aims to investigate and compare the toxic effects of four types of metal oxide (ZnO, TiO$_2$, SiO$_2$ and Al$_2$O$_3$) nanoparticles with similar primary size ($\sim$20 nm) on human fetal lung fibroblasts (HFL1) *in vitro*. METHODS: The HFL1 cells were exposed to the nanoparticles, and toxic effects were analyzed by using MTT assay, cellular morphology observation and Hoechst 33 258 staining. RESULTS: The results show that the four types of metal oxide nanoparticles lead to cellular mitochondrial dysfunction, morphological modifications and apoptosis at the concentration range of 0.25-1.50 mg/mL and the toxic effects are obviously displayed in dose-dependent manner. ZnO is the most toxic nanomaterials followed by TiO$_2$, SiO$_2$, and Al$_2$O$_3$ nanoparticles in a descending order. CONCLUSION: The results highlight the differential cytotoxicity associated with exposure to ZnO, TiO$_2$, SiO$_2$, and Al$_2$O$_3$ nanoparticles, and suggest an extreme attention to safety utilization of these nanomaterials.

Keywords: metal oxide nanoparticles; toxic effects; fibroblasts

Biomed. Environ. Sci., *2011*, *24*(6): *661-669.*

55. 子宫内炎症增加小鼠妊娠期间金纳米粒子的母胎转移具有尺寸依赖性

Intrauterine inflammation increases materno-fetal transfer of gold nanoparticles in a size-dependent manner in murine pregnancy

Abstract：The materno-fetal transfer of nanoparticles is a critical issue in designing theranoustic nanoparticles for in vivo applications during pregnancy. Recent studies have reported that certain nanoparticles can cross the placental barrier in healthy pregnant animals depending on the size and surface modification of the nanoparticles and the developmental stages of the fetuses. However, materno-fetal transfer under pathological pregnant conditions has not been examined so far. Here, it is shown that intrauterine inflammation can enhance the materno-fetal transfer of nanoparticles in the late gestation stage of murine pregnancy in a size-dependent manner. Three different-sized gold nanoparticles (Au NPs) with diameters of 3 (Au3), 13 (Au13) and 32 (Au32) nm are applied. The accumulation of Au3 and Au13 nanoparticles in the fetuses is significantly increased in intrauterine inflammatory mice compared with healthy control mice：the concentration of Au3 is much higher than Au13 in fetal tissues of intrauterine inflammatory mice. In contrast, Au32 nanoparticles cannot cross the placental barrier either in healthy or in intrauterine inflammatory mice. The possible underlying mechanism of the increased materno-fetal transfer of small-sized nanoparticles on pathological conditions is inferred to be the structural and functional abnormalities of the placenta under intrauterine inflammation. The size of the nanoparticles is one of the critical factors which determines the extent of fetal exposure to nanoparticles in murine pregnancy under inflammatory conditions.

Keywords：gold nanoparticles；pregnancy；materno-fetal transfer；intrauterine inflammation；nanosafety

Small, 2013, *9*：2432-2439.

56. 孕龄和表面修饰在小鼠妊娠期间对纳米颗粒母胎转移的影响

Effects of gestational age and surface modification on materno-fetal transfer of nanoparticles in murine pregnancy

Abstract：Nanoparticle exposure in pregnancy may result in placental damage and fetotoxicity; however, the factors that determine fetal nanoparticle exposure are unclear. Here we have assessed the effect of gestational age and nanoparticle composition on fetal accumulation of maternally-administered nanomaterials in mice. We determined the placental and fetal uptake of 13 nm gold nanoparticles with different surface modifications (ferritin, PEG and citrate) following intravenous administration at E5. 5-15. 5. We showed that prior to E11. 5, all tested nanoparticles could be visualized and detected in fetal tissues in significant amounts; however, fetal gold levels declined dramatically post-E11. 5. In contrast, Au-nanoparticle accumulation in the extraembryonic tissues (EET) increased 6-15 fold with gestational age. Fetal and EET accumulation of ferritin- and PEG-modified nanoparticles was considerably greater than citrate-capped nanoparticles. No signs of toxicity were observed. Fetal exposure to nanoparticles in murine pregnancy is, therefore, influenced by both stage of embryonic/placental maturation and nanoparticle surface composition.

Sci. Rep., *2012*, *2*：*847*.

57. 纳米安全性需要关注内分泌系统的研究

Nanotoxicity: A growing need for study in the endocrine system

Abstract: Nanomaterials (NMs) are engineered for commercial purposes such as semiconductors, building materials, cosmetics, and drug carriers, while natural nanoparticles (NPs) already exist in the environment. Due to their unique physicochemical properties, they may interact actively with biological systems. Some of these interactions might be detrimental to human health, and therefore studies on the potential 'nanotoxicity' of these materials in different organ systems are warranted. The purpose of developing the concept of nanotoxicity is to recognize and evaluate the hazards and risks of NMs and evaluate safety. This review will summarize and discuss recent reports derived from cell lines or animal models concerning the effects of NMs on, and their application in, the endocrine system of mammalian and other species. It will present an update on current studies of the effects of some typical NMs—such as metal-based NMs, carbon-based NMs, and dendrimers—on endocrine functions, in which some effects are adverse or unwanted and others are favorable or intended. Disruption of endocrine function is associated with adverse health outcomes including reproductive failure, metabolic syndrome, and some types of cancer. Further investigations are therefore required to obtain a thorough understanding of any potential risk of pathological endocrine disruption from products containing NMs. This review aims to provide impetus for further studies on the interactions of NMs with endocrine functions.

Small, 2013, *9(9-10)*: *1654-1671*.

58. 气管灌注纳米氧化铈后的肺沉积和肺外转移

Lung deposition and extrapulmonary translocation of nano-ceria after intratracheal instillation

Abstract: The broad potential applications of manufactured nanomaterials call for urgent assessment of their environmental and biological safety. However, most of the previous work focused on the cell level performance; little was known about the consequences of nanomaterial exposure at the whole-body and organ levels. In the present paper, the radiotracer technique was employed to study the pulmonary deposition and the translocation to secondary target organs after ceria nanoparticles (nano-ceria) were intratracheally instilled into Wistar rats. It was found that 63.9% +/−8.2% of the instilled nano-ceria remained in the lung by 28 d postexposure and the elimination half-life was 103 d. At the end of the test period, only 1/8-1/3 of the daily elimination of nano-ceria from the lung was cleared via the gastrointestinal tract, suggesting that phagocytosis by alveolar macrophages (AMs) with subsequent removal towards the larynx was no longer the predominant route for the elimination of nano-ceria from the lung. The whole-body redistribution of nano-ceria demonstrated that the deposited nano-ceria could penetrate through the alveolar wall into the systemic circulation and accumulate in the extrapulmonary organs. In vitro study suggested that nano-ceria would agglomerate and form sediments in the bronchoalveolar aqueous surrounding while binding to protein would be conducive to the redispersion of nano-ceria. The decrease in the size of agglomerates might enhance the penetration of nano-ceria into the systemic circulation. Our findings suggested that the effect of nanomaterial exposure, even at low concentration, should be assessed because of the potential lung and systemic cumulative toxicity of the nanomaterials.

Nanotechnology, 2010, 21(28): 285103.

59. 改变暴露媒介可以逆转纳米氧化铈颗粒对大肠杆菌的细胞毒性

Changing exposure media can reverse the cytotoxicity of ceria nanoparticles for *Escherichia coli*.

Abstract：Ceria nanoparticles have attracted a great deal of concern about their impact on human health and the environment due to their widespread applications. In the present work, different exposure media (normal saline and phosphate-buffered saline [PBS]) were used to adjust the surface charge density in order to investigate the influence of surface charge on the cytotoxicity of ceria nanoparticles for Escherichia coli. The results showed that the direct contact mediated by the electrostatic attraction between the cell wall and the positive-charged ceria nanoparticles in normal saline would result in outer membrane destabilization, increased reactive oxygen species (ROS) production and loss of viability. The situation in PBS was totally different, with significantly reduced contacts, so no outer membrane destabilization, no increased ROS production, and no cytotoxicity. The results suggested that surface charge density was closely involved in the cytotoxicity of ceria nanoparticles for E. coli. This work as a well designed comparison study contributes to a better understanding of the charge-associated biological effects of nanomaterials.

Keywords：ceria nanoparticles; cytotoxicity; exposure media; surface charge density; in situ assessment

Nanotoxicology, 2012, 6(3)：233-240.

60. La₂O₃ 纳米颗粒对陆生植物黄瓜的药害及其在体内的生物转化

Phytotoxicity and biotransformation of La₂O₃ nanoparticles in a terrestrial plant cucumber (Cucumis sativus).

Abstract: With the increasing applications of metal-based nanoparticles in various commercial products, it is necessary to address their environmental fate and potential toxicity. In this work, we assessed the phytotoxicity of lanthanum oxide (La₂O₃) NPs to cucumber plants and determined its distribution and biotransformation in roots by TEM and EDS, as well as STXM and NEXAFS. LaCl₃ was also studied as a reference toxicant. La₂O₃ NPs and LaCl₃ were both transformed to needle-like LaPO₄ nanoclusters in the intercellular regions of the cucumber roots. In vitro experiments demonstrated that the dissolution of La₂O₃ NPs was significantly enhanced by acetic acid. Accordingly, we proposed that the dissolution of NPs at the root surface induced by the organic acids extruded from root cells played an important role in the phytotoxicity of La₂O₃ NPs. The reactions of active NPs at the nano-bio interface should be taken into account when studying the toxicity of dissolvable metal-based nanoparticles.

Keywords: La₂O₃ nanoparticles, phytotoxicity, dissolution, biotransformation

Nanotoxicology, 2011, 5(4): 743-753.

61. 纳米稀土氧化物对植物根伸展的影响
Effects of rare earth oxide nanoparticles on root elongation of plants

Abstract: The phytotoxicity of four rare earth oxide nanoparticles, nano-CeO_2, nano-La_2O_3, nano-Gd_2O_3 and nano-Yb_2O_3 on seven higher plant species (radish, rape, tomato, lettuce, wheat, cabbage, and cucumber) were investigated in the present study by means of root elongation experiments. Their effects on root growth varied greatly between different nanoparticles and plant species. A suspension of 2000 mg L^{-1} nano-CeO_2 had no effect on the root elongation of six plants, except lettuce. On the contrary, 2000 mg L^{-1} suspensions of nano-La_2O_3, nano-Gd_2O_3 and nano-Yb_2O_3 severely inhibited the root elongation of all the seven species. Inhibitory effects of nano-La_2O_3, nano-Gd_2O_3, and nano-Yb_2O_3 also differed in the different growth process of plants. For wheat, the inhibition mainly took place during the seed incubation process, while lettuce and rape were inhibited on both seed soaking and incubation process. The fifty percent inhibitory concentrations (IC_{50}) for rape were about 40 mg L^{-1} of nano-La_2O_3, 20mg L^{-1} of nano-Gd_2O_3, and 70 mg L^{-1} of nano-Yb_2O_3, respectively. In the concentration ranges used in this study, the RE^{3+} ion released from the nanoparticles had negligible effects on the root elongation. These results are helpful in understanding phytotoxicity of rare earth oxide nanoparticles.

Keywords: rare earth oxide; nanoparticles; phytotoxicity; root elongation; toxicity effects

Chemosphere, 2010, 78(3): 273-279.

62. 表面化学设计制备低毒安全的纳米材料，碳纳米管，富勒烯，金属富勒烯和石墨烯

Low-toxic and safe nanomaterials by surface-chemical design, carbon nanotubes, fullerenes, metallofullerenes, and graphenes.

Abstract: The toxicity grade for a bulk material can be approximately determined by three factors (chemical composition, dose, and exposure route). However, for a nanomaterial it depends on more than ten factors. Interestingly, some nano-factors (like huge surface adsorbability, small size, etc.) that endow nanomaterials with new biomedical functions are also potential causes leading to toxicity or damage to the living organism. Is it possible to create safe nanomaterials if such a number of complicated factors need to be regulated? We herein try to find answers to this important question. We first discuss chemical processes that are applicable for nanosurface modifications, in order to improve biocompatibility, regulate ADME, and reduce the toxicity of carbon nanomaterials (carbon nanotubes, fullerenes, metallofullerenes, and graphenes). Then the biological/toxicological effects of surface-modified and unmodified carbon nanomaterials are comparatively discussed from two aspects: the lowered toxic responses or the enhanced biomedical functions. We summarize the eight biggest challenges in creating low-toxicity and safer nanomaterials and some significant topics of future research needs: to find out safer nanofactors; to establish controllable surface modifications and simpler chemistries for low-toxic nanomaterials; to explore the nanotoxicity mechanisms; to justify the validity of current toxicological theories in nanotoxicology; to create standardized nanomaterials for toxicity tests; to build theoretical models for cellular and molecular interactions of nanoparticles; and to establish systematical knowledge frameworks for nanotoxicology.

Nanoscale, 2011, 3(2): 362-382.

63. 纳米材料产生毒性的化学机制:生成细胞内活性氧

Chemical mechanisms of the toxicological properties of nanomaterials: Generation of intracellular reactive oxygen species

Abstract: As more and more nanomaterials with novel physicochemical properties or new functions are created and used in different research fields and industrial sectors, the scientific and public concerns about their toxic effects on human health and the environment are also growing quickly. In the past decade, the study of the toxicological properties of nanomaterials/nanoparticles has formed a new research field: nanotoxicology. However, most of the data published relate to toxicological phenomena and there is less understanding of the underlying mechanism for nanomaterial-induced toxicity. Nanomaterial-induced reactive oxygen species (ROS) play a key role in cellular and tissue toxicity. Herein, we classify the pathways for intracellular ROS production by nanomaterials into 1) the direct generation of ROS through nanomaterial-catalyzed free-radical reactions in cells, and 2) the indirect generation of ROS through disturbing the inherent biochemical equilibria in cells. We also discuss the chemical mechanisms associated with above pathways of intracellular ROS generation, from the viewpoint of the high reactivity of atoms on the nanosurface. We hope to aid in the understanding of the chemical origin of nanotoxicity to provide new insights for chemical and material scientists for the rational design and creation of safer and greener nanomaterials.

Keywords: nanoparticles; oxygen; reactive intermediates; reaction mechanisms; toxicity

Chem. Asian J., *2013*, *8*: *2342-2353*.

附录 2　中英文术语对照表

中文术语	英文表述	定义
纳米尺度	Nanoscale	处于 1～100 nm 之间的尺寸范围。
纳米材料	Nanomaterial	任一外部维度、内部或表面结构处于纳米尺度的材料。
纳米物体	Nano-object	一维、二维或三维外部维度处于纳米尺度的物体。 注：用于所有相互分离的纳米尺度物体的通用术语。
纳米结构	Nanostructure	一个或多个部分处于纳米尺度区域的相互关联的组成部分。 注：区域由性质不连续的边界来界定。
纳米技术	Nanotechnology	应用科学知识操纵和控制纳米尺度的物质以利用与单个原子、分子或块体材料性质显著不同的、与尺寸和结构相关的性质和现象。
工程纳米颗粒	Engineered nanoparticle	为了特定目的或功能而设计的纳米材料。
纳米颗粒	Nanoparticle	直径（例如几何、气动、流动性、投影面积或其他参数）小于 100 nm 的颗粒，或三个维度都处于纳米尺度的颗粒。 注：如果纳米材料最长轴与最短轴的长度差异显著时，可被称为纳米棒和纳米盘，差异大于三倍时称为"显著"。
纳米气溶胶	Nanoaerosol	由纳米颗粒及纳米结构颗粒构成的气溶胶。
石墨烯	Graphene	从石墨材料中剥离出的单层碳原子面材料，是碳的二维结构，属于复式六角晶格。
碳纳米管	Carbon nanotube	由碳构成的纳米管。 注：通常指由石墨烯片层卷曲而成的无缝管，分为单壁碳纳米管（或称单层碳纳米管）和多壁碳纳米管（或称多层碳纳米管）。
富勒烯	Fullerene	具有多于 20 个碳原子所构成的三维排列的碳原子闭合笼状结构。 注：具有 60 个碳原子（C_{60}）的闭合笼状结构被称为富勒烯。
量子点	Quantum dot	把导带电子、价带空穴及激子在三个空间方向上束缚住的半导体纳米结构。
气相二氧化硅	Fumed silica	热解生产的以粉体形式存在的二氧化硅，其中含有的颗粒处于纳米尺度。

续表

中文术语	英文表述	定义
纳米簇	Nanocluster	非共价或共价键连接的原子或分子,最大外形尺寸通常处于纳米尺度。
纳米复合材料	Nanocomposite	多相结构,其中至少一个相的一维尺寸处于纳米尺度。
纳米晶体	Nanocrystal	由原子、离子或分子以周期性晶格形式构成的纳米尺度固体。
纳米纤维	Nanofibre	有韧性、能弯曲的纳米棒(nanorod)。
纳米盘	Nanoplate	其中一维的外部尺寸处于纳米尺度,其他两个外部尺寸显著增大的纳米结构。 注1:纳米板最小的外部尺寸是厚度。 注2:尺寸差异至少是3倍。 注3:较大外部尺寸不一定在纳米尺度。
纳米线	Nanowire	具有在横向上被限制在 100 nm 以下(纵向没有限制)的一维结构。
树枝状	Dendrimer	由重复增长反应合成,从一个单体建立起来的三维大分子,新的分支逐步添加,直至形成一个对称分支结构。 注:完美的分支被称为树枝状,而不完美的分支被称为超支化(hyperbranched)。
初级颗粒	Primary particle	不是由其他颗粒组成的颗粒。 注:通常指凝结发生之前,在气相成核阶段形成的颗粒。
次级颗粒	Secondary particle	通过气相化学反应形成的颗粒(气体到颗粒变化)。
超细颗粒	Ultrafine particle	当量直径小于 100 nm 的颗粒物。

附录 3 生产与工作场所纳米颗粒暴露
监测与评估案例

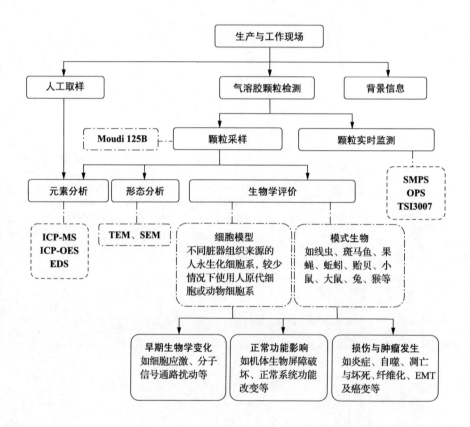

附录 4 典型现场暴露监测文献数据汇编

参考文献	纳米材料种类	生产现场	生产活动	指标和仪器	背景	电镜样品
Tsai et al. 2009a[119]	alumina silver	research lab, effectiveness of fume hood tested	pouring transferring	NSD; FMPS Morphology: SEM and STEM Element comp: EDX	1 m in front of fume hood, before each experiment, subtraction from source concentration	on copper grids in sampler of own design
Tsai et al. 2009b[120]	CNT	research lab	synthesis by CVD	NSD: APS, FMPS Morphology: TEM, SEM Elemental comp: EDX	1 m away from fume hood, before, during and after each operation	on copper grids in sampler of own design
Brouwer et al. 2009[121]	fumed silica	production of toner and printing inks industry	bag-emptying	NC: ELPI NSD: SMPS Active surface area: DC (LQ1) Morphology: TEM Element comp: EDX	CPC in an adjacent room non-activity	on TEM grids by personal air sampling
Bello et al. 2009[20]	CNT composite	research lab	dry and wet phase abrasive machining (band-saw and rotary cutting wheel)	NC: CPC, FMPS, APS NSD: FMPS, APS Surface area: calculated MC: DustTrack Respirable fibres: NIOSH method 7400 Morphology and particle size: TEM Element comp: EDX	before activity, shown as reference, some results corrected	on Cu grid using thermophoretic and electrostatic precipitators

续表

参考文献	纳米材料种类	生产现场	生产活动	指标和仪器	背景	电镜样品
Park et al. 2009[84]	Ag	commercial production facility	liquid-phase process (batch reaction, filtering, drying, grinding)	NSD: SMPS Surface area, components, Morphology: TEM	pre activity, subtraction	electrostatic precipitator on TEM grids
Demou et al. 2009[32]	NaCl $BiPO_4$ $CaSO_4$ Bi_2O_3 TiO_2 SiO_2 WO_3 Cu/ZnO Cu/SiO_2 Cu/ZrO_2 Ta_2O_5/SiO_2 $Pt/Ba/Al_2O_3$	research lab	synthesis via FSP, collecting product	NC: CPC NSD: SMPS MC: DustTrack (PM1), SidePak (PM10)	on no activity days, pre and post activity, used to normalise measurement data	
Peters et al. 2008[33]	lithium titanate metal oxide	industrial	wet mill spray drier rotary calciner	NC: CPC, OPC MC: filter samples, estimates from CPC, OPC Elemental analysis: ICP-AES Morphology, composition: TEM		mixed cellulose ester filters
Möhlmann et al. 2009[122]	ZnO SiO_2 silanes	not mentioned	mixing of powder with liquid binder, powder filled into an oven, spraying, flame spraying	NC: CPC NSD: SMPS, APS MSD: personl air samplers MC of respirable and inhalable: static dust sampler Morphology: TEM, SEM	not addressed	

续表

参考文献	纳米材料种类	生产现场	生产活动	指标和仪器	背景	电镜样品
Manodori et al. 2009[123]	nanofillers	research lab	deposition of films by PECVD and PVD, compounding of polymers	NC: CPC NSD: WRAS	not addressed	
Plitzko S 2009[124]	TiO_2, nanofibers, ceramic nanopowder	research lab and small scale industry	synthesis, processing	NC: SMPS, CPC NSD: WRAS MC: aerosol spectrometer Morphology: SEM Elemental comp: EDX	preferably during night	gold filters or thermal precipitator
Bae et al. 2010[125]	metal nanopowder （Al, Cu, Cu/Ni alloy）		synthesis (wire electrical explosion process)	NC: CPC NSD: SMPS		
Johnson et al. 2010[76]	carbon nanomaterials, CNT and fullerenes	Research lab	a) transfer of CNMs from storage containers to weighing balance b) sonication	NC: HHPC-6 hand held particle counter, CPC Morphology: TEM Elemental comp: EDX	inside lab before task, subtracted from process-specific measurements	filter based air sampling
Methner et al. 2010[38]	CNT, CNF, carbon nanopearls, fullerenes, TiO_2, CuO, Ag, Mn, Co-oxides, Fe-oxides, Al, Si-Fe, quantum dots	research lab to industrial production	synthesis, handling (weighing, mixing, sonication etc.), production of composite	NC: CPC, OPC MC: filter Morphology: TEM Elemental comp: EDX	same room but away	filter samples

续表

参考文献	纳米材料种类	生产现场	生产活动	指标和仪器	背景	电镜样品
Wang et al. 2010[126]	carbon black	industrial site	pelletizing, packaging, warehouse	NSD: SMPS, MEAD; SAC: NSAM, MEAD	outdoor, upwind and indoors prior to activity (not all sites)	
Tsai et al. 2010[36]	Al_2O_3	research lab (fume hood)	manual transfer, pouring	NSD: FMPS, APS	1 m in front of hood, before tasks, subtracted from results	
Evans et al. 2010[127]	CNF	industrial	production, mixing, drying, thermal treatment	NC: CPC; NSD: ELPI, FPSS; MC (respirable): photometer (DustTrack); Active surface area: diffusion charger; Photoelectric response: photoelectric aerosol sensor		
Cena et al. 2011[42]	CNT	production facility	weighing, sanding of CNT reinforced epoxy samples	NC: CPC, OPC; MC (respirable): OPC; Morphology: TEM	prior to process in glove box, process to background ratios calculated	on copper grids in sampler of own design
van Broekhuizen et al. 2011[72]	TiO_2 (anatase) silica	outdoor working	filling spraying system and spraying a liquid window coating, applying a cement repair mortar to a bridge, mixing of cement repair mortar, nano-concrete drilling	NC, number-averaged particle diameter, surface area: Aerasense (NanoTracer)	at workplace preceding the activities and Near-field emissions (within 1-2 metres)	

续表

参考文献	纳米材料种类	生产现场	生产活动	指标和仪器	背景	电镜样品
Fleury et al. 2013[128]	CNT	small-scale pilot line	weighing, mixing, grinding of composite	NSD: ELPI, SMPS Morphology: TEM Elemental comp: EDX		VTT aspiration sampler
Ogura et al. 2011[129]	SiC, LiFePO$_4$, ZnO	industrial manufacturing plant	synthesis, collection, bagging	NC: CPC, OPC NSD: ELPI Morphology: SEM	prior to activity, outdoors or far from working area	filter (Nuclepore)
Wang et al. 2011[130]	Si; CNT	pilot, industrial	synthesis, collection, bagging, packaging, cleaning, production of composites	NC: CPC NSD: FMPS, SMPS Surface area: NSAM NC, SAC, volume distribution: UNPA (universal nanoparticle analyser)	outside production facility	
Tsai et al. 2011[131]	SiO$_2$, carbon black, CaCO$_3$	industrial	mixing, bagging, manufacturing	NC,NSD: SMPS MC (respirable): cyclone MSD: MOUDI Elemental analysis: filters by ICP-OES, UV-Vis	outside	
Lee et al. 2011[132]	TiO$_2$, Ag	research, industrial	production, collection	NSD: SMPS, dust monitor MC: filter samples Morphology: TEM Elemental analysis: ICP-MS from filters, EDX		from filter samples

续表

参考文献	纳米材料种类	生产现场	生产活动	指标和仪器	背景	电镜样品
Leppänen et al. 2012[133]	CeO_2	industrial	flame spray process used for coating	NC: CPC, ELPI NSD: SMPS, ELPI MC: ELPI, TEOM Morphology: SEM, TEM Elemental comp: EDX	prior and post activity	VTT aspiration sampler, electrostatic precipitator
R'Mili et al. 2011[134]	CNT	industrial	pouring, shoveling	Real-time elemental comp: LIBS Morphology: SEM, TEM Elemental comp: EDX		VTT aspiration sampler, VTT diffusion sampler
van Broekhuizen et al. 2012[135]	nanomaterial not revealed in all cases, TiO_2, $CaCO_3$, talc, ZnO, Al_2O_3	industrial settings	electroplating plant-dipping + abrasion, nanopaint manufacturing-opening bags + mixing, pigment manufacturing-mixing, production of non-reflective glass-cutting + breaking, manufacturing of fluorescent tubes-mixing, coating, finishing (polishing, high T) car refinishing-abrasion + spraying	NC, number-averaged particle diameter, surface area; Aerasense (NanoTracer)	before activities	

续表

参考文献	纳米材料种类	生产现场	生产活动	指标和仪器	背景	电镜样品
Wang et al. 2012[136]	Si	pilot-scale facility	synthesis, collection, bagging, cleaning	NC: CPC NSD: FMPS, SMPS Surface area: NSAM Morphology: SEM Elemental comp: EDX	outside production enclosure, during night when no activity	Nanometer Aerosol Sampler
Ham, et al. 2012[137]	TiO₂, Al, Ag, Cu	ENM workplace, welding site	ENM manufacturing, welding	NC: P-Trak model 8525 NSD: SMPS 3936 L75 SAC: AeroTrak model 9000 MC: aerosol spectrometer Grimm 1.109 (<1 μm particles); filter samples Morphology: SEM Composition: EDS	Time-activity diary (TAD) to record contextual information, background basically during night (no operation)	From PTFE filters

注: Mass Concentration (MC),质量浓度;Mass Size Distribution (MSD),质量尺寸分布;Particle Number Concentration (NC),颗粒数量浓度;Particle Number Size Distribution (NSD),颗粒数量尺寸分布;Surface Area Concentration (SAC),表面积浓度

附录 5 监测仪器分类汇编

度量标准	设备	附注
质量浓度	水平重力式多段分级采样器	阶式撞击采样器切割粒径约 100 nm（Berner 型低压撞击，或微孔撞击）。可进行质量和化学成分分析。
	锥形元件振荡微量天平（TEOM）	灵敏的实时监测设备，如锥形元件振荡微量天平（TEOM），可用于实时在线检测一定尺寸范围的纳米气溶胶质量浓度。
	扫描电迁移粒径谱仪（SMPS）	根据气溶胶颗粒在电场中的迁移率不同，得到气溶胶尺寸分布及数量浓度。当颗粒形状和密度是已知的或假定时，数据可被转换成气溶胶质量浓度。
	静电低压撞击器（ELPI™）	将气溶胶颗粒按空气动力学直径的大小分段顺序收集，得到颗粒物尺寸分布。已知颗粒物的电荷和密度，则可计算出颗粒物的质量浓度。
数量浓度	凝聚核粒子计数器（CPC）	CPC 可以实时检测的颗粒物数量浓度。它不具有对纳米颗粒进行尺寸分级的功能。P-Trak 检测上限为 $1\ \mu m$。
	扫描电迁移粒径谱仪（SMPS）	根据气溶胶颗粒在电场中的迁移率不同，得到气溶胶尺寸分布及数量浓度。
	静电低压撞击器（ELPI™）	将气溶胶颗粒按空气动力学直径的大小分段顺序收集，得到颗粒物尺寸分布，可作为数量浓度。尺寸分级采样器也可进行离线分析。
	光学粒子计数器	不能检测粒径小于 300 nm 的颗粒，不适用于纳米颗粒检测。
	电子显微镜	离线分析电子显微镜样品可提供气溶胶数量浓度的尺寸分布信息。
表面积浓度	扫描电迁移粒径谱仪（SMPS）	根据气溶胶颗粒在电场中的迁移率不同，得到气溶胶尺寸分布及数量浓度。在某些情况下，数量浓度可以转换成表面面积浓度。
	静电低压撞击器（ELPI™）	将气溶胶颗粒按空气动力学直径的大小分段顺序收集。颗粒物粒径大于 100 nm，活性表面积与几何表面积不成比例。
	SMPS 和 ELPI™ 联合使用	测量空气动力学和迁移率的不同能够用于推测不规则形状颗粒的大小，能够更进一步的估算表面积。
	单极电晕器	实时检测气溶胶活性表面积。颗粒物粒径大于 100 nm，活性表面积与几何表面积不成比例。值得注意的是并不是所有的市售单极电晕器都能检测出粒径小于 100 nm 的颗粒活性表面积。如果采用合适的预分离器，单极电晕器适用于纳米颗粒。
	电子显微镜	离线分析电子显微镜样品可提供颗粒表面积浓度信息，还可提供颗粒投影面积信息，与颗粒几何面积相关。

附录 6 暴露现场检测数据记录表

现场检测记录总表

No.

序号	日期	地点	检测阶段	文档号	检测人	复核

第二阶段(S2)检测原始信息表　　　　　　　　　　　文档号：＿＿＿＿＿＿＿

记录表序号	地点	仪器	防护措施	
测量位置与过程		背景值1 (P/cm³)	背景值1 (P/cm³)	背景值1 (P/cm³)	备注
测量位置与过程		测量值	测量值	测量值	备注
测量位置与过程		测量值	测量值	测量值	备注
测量位置与过程		测量值	测量值	测量值	备注
测量位置与过程		测量值	测量值	测量值	备注

S2 检测结果汇总表　　　　　　　　　　　　　　　　文档号：_____

文档号	释放源辨识	背景值 (P/cm³)	释放值 (P/cm³)	显著性	是否转入 第三阶段(S3)

第三阶段(S3)检测原始信息表-1　　　　　　　　　　　　　　　　　文档号：＿＿＿＿＿＿＿

S3 检测流程	
检测编号	
项目名称	
项目代码	
检测方法	
检测对象 （三个可选项）	□富勒烯（C_{60}） □单壁碳纳米管（SWCNTs） □多壁碳纳米管（MWCNTs） □银纳米颗粒 □铁纳米颗粒 □二氧化钛 □氧化铝 □氧化铈 □氧化锌 □二氧化硅 □树状大分子 □纳米黏土 □金纳米颗粒 □纳米颗粒混合物 □其他：＿＿＿＿＿
检测人员	
检测开始日期	＿＿＿：＿＿＿＿：＿＿＿＿＿（年：月：日）
检测结束日期	＿＿＿：＿＿＿＿：＿＿＿＿＿（年：月：日）
数据使用范围	□所有的项目合作者 □从＿＿＿：＿＿＿：＿＿＿＿（年：月：日）允许项目合作者使用 □只有经授权后才可使用数据 □只针对研究所开放 □无有效数据
监测日期	：＿＿＿＿＿：＿＿＿＿＿＿（年：月：日）

S3 级检测原始信息表-2　　　　　　　　　　　　　　　　　文档号：＿＿＿＿＿＿

检测方信息	
检测编号	
检测名称	
单位名称、地址、联系人及联系方式	
检测人员	
备注	

检测场所信息	
检测编号	
检测场所名称、地址	
工作区域面积	
采样地点，与释放源距离	
生产活动记录	
工作人员数量(位)	
工作时间(小时)	
管理经验	□弱 □默认级别 □较好的管理经验 □有效的内务管理 □全封闭过程
检测场所补充描述	

S3 检测原始信息表-3   文档号：_____

检测仪器信息表				
检测编号				
仪器名称	仪器型号	品牌	用途	备注

S3 检测原始信息表-4　　　　　　　　　　　　　　　　　　文档号：＿＿＿＿＿＿＿＿

现场工人信息	
检测编号	
工人数量（位）	□工作间：＿＿＿＿ □室内：＿＿＿＿ □室外：＿＿＿＿
工人职位	
生产培训及经验	□受训 ＋ 经验丰富 □受训 ＋ 经验不足 □未受训 ＋ 经验丰富 □未受训 ＋ 经验不足
工人是否衣着整洁	□是 □否 □不适用

工人是否了解	纳米材料的危险性	□是 □否
	存储	□是 □否 □不适用
	维护	□是 □否 □不适用

备注	

S3 检测原始信息表-5　　　　　　　　　　　　　　　　　文档号：＿＿＿＿＿＿＿

通风设施		
检测编号		
通风方式	□不通风 □自然通风-打开门和窗户 □自然通风-门和窗户关闭 □机械通风-输入及排出空气 □机械通风-仅输入空气 □机械通风-仅排出空气	
通风系统效能	□弱 □一般 □高	
每小时的空气变化		
机械通风是否使用过滤器	□是 □否	
过滤器分类	□计重过滤器	□G1 □G2 □G3 □G4
	□除尘效率过滤器	□F5 □F6 □F7 □F8 □F9
	□HEPA 过滤器	□H10 □H11 □H12 □H13 □H14
	□ULPA 过滤器	□U15 □U16 □U17
空气再循环	□否 □是	

续表

通风设施	
隔离说明（如适用）	□不隔离 □部分隔离,不通风 □部分隔离,通风 □完全隔离,没有排气通风 □完全隔离,排气通风,空气不流通
暴露控制的时间（秒）	开始：＿＿＿：＿＿＿：＿＿ 结束：＿＿＿：＿＿＿：＿＿
通风口气流速度	＿＿＿＿＿＿＿ 米/秒
生产现场空气流速	＿＿＿＿＿＿＿ 米/秒
室内气压	＿＿＿＿＿＿＿ 米/秒
平均相对湿度	＿＿＿＿＿＿＿ ％
温度	＿＿＿℃
风向	□下风口（从释放源到工人） □上风口（从工人到释放源）
备注	

S3 检测原始信息表-6   文档号：＿＿＿＿＿＿

防护信息		
检测编号		
工人换班时间	开始：＿＿：＿＿：＿ 结束：＿：＿＿：＿	
隔离/个人防护	□不隔离 □部分隔离不通风 □部分隔离通风 □完全隔离不通风 □完全隔离通风	
工人暴露时间		
呼吸防护设备及型号	□呼吸器/过滤面罩	型号：
	□呼吸器/半面罩,微粒过滤器	型号：
	□呼吸器/全面罩,微粒过滤器	型号：
	□电动送风过滤式呼吸器半或全脸面具	型号：
	□电动送风过滤式呼吸器头盔或头罩	型号：
	□呼吸器/空气恒流与压缩空气供应	型号：
	□呼吸器/空气恒流	型号：
	□呼吸器/半面罩/需求阀 BA(气流或自足)	型号：
	□呼吸器/全面罩/需求阀 BA(气流或独立),正压	型号：
	□呼吸器/全面罩/需求阀 BA(气流或独立),负压	型号：
护目镜/眼镜	□无 □护目镜,眼镜 □护目镜,4 型抗粉尘 □护目镜,5 型抗气体,烟雾,气溶胶 □安装到头盔上的眼睛防护罩	
佩戴者是否使用光学眼镜	□是 □否	
工人是否佩戴	头盔	□是 □否
	面罩	□是 □否

防护信息	
听力保护	□否 □听力保护,耳塞 □听力防护,耳套 □头盔上附带的耳罩
防护套装类型	□无 □非保护性工作服 □套装,型号:_____ □其他:
手套类型	□无 □手套（化学型） □手套（机械型） □手套（对热和火焰的防护） □其他:
备注	

S3 检测原始信息表-7　　　　　　　　　　　　　　　　　文档号：＿＿＿＿＿＿

产品信息	
检测编号	
产品铭牌	
制造商/进口商名称	
是否纳米尺度材料	□是 □否
产品形态	□液体 □粉末 □固体 □纤维 □膏状
材料纯度	□100% □配料
产品黏度	□低黏度 □中等黏度 □高黏度
化学式	
材料密度	＿＿＿＿ g/cm³
密度类型	□体积 □元素 □聚集
产品含尘类型	□硬颗粒 □颗粒状,片状或丸状 □粗尘 □细尘 □极精细粉
含尘检测系统	
粉尘量	＿＿＿＿＿＿＿＿ mg/kg
水分含量	□干品（水分含量<5%） □5%～10% 水分含量 □>10% 水分含量

产品信息	
产品的分子质量	＿＿＿＿＿＿＿ g/mol
BET 表面积	＿＿＿＿＿＿＿ m^2/g
体积比表面积	＿＿＿＿＿＿＿ m^2/m^3
原始粒径	＿＿＿＿＿＿＿ nm
包被	□是 □否
兴奋剂	□是 □否
产品备注	

S3 检测原始信息表-8　　　　　　　　　　　　　　　文档号：＿＿＿＿＿＿

检测采样总表	
检测编号	
检测日期	＿＿＿：＿＿＿＿：＿＿＿＿＿＿（年：月：日）
检测地点名称	
工人数量	
检测地点空气速度	＿＿＿＿＿ 米/秒

在线检测设备				
设备名称与序列号	检测地点描述	采样的时间(时：分：秒)和采样信息		设置
装置 1	□背景，近场方法 □背景，远场方法 □活动，个人 □活动，静态，距离 ＿＿ 米	开始：＿＿＿：＿＿＿：＿＿＿ 结束：＿＿＿：＿＿＿：＿＿＿ 抽检情况 □随机 □典型 □顺序	采样规范 □个人 □静态 □活动 □固定	采样时间 = ＿＿＿ 秒 流速 = ＿＿＿＿＿ 升/分钟 稀释＿＿＿＿＿ 冲击 ＿＿＿＿＿ 与释放源距离＿＿＿＿＿ 米
装置 2	□背景，近场方法 □背景，远场方法 □活动，个人 □活动，静态，距离 ＿＿ 米	开始：＿＿＿：＿＿＿：＿＿＿ 结束：＿＿＿：＿＿＿：＿＿＿ 抽检情况 □随机 □典型 □顺序	采样规范 □个人 □静态 □活动 □固定	采样时间 = ＿＿＿ 秒 流速 = ＿＿＿＿＿ 升/分钟 稀释＿＿＿＿＿ 冲击 ＿＿＿＿＿ 与释放源距离＿＿＿＿＿ 米
装置 3	□背景，近场方法 □背景，远场方法 □活动，个人 □活动，静态，距离 ＿＿ 米	开始：＿＿＿：＿＿＿：＿＿＿ 结束：＿＿＿：＿＿＿：＿＿＿ 抽检情况 □随机 □典型 □顺序	采样规范 □个人 □静态 □活动 □固定	采样时间 = ＿＿＿ 秒 流速 = ＿＿＿＿＿ 升/分钟 稀释＿＿＿＿＿ 冲击＿＿＿＿＿ 与释放源距离＿＿＿＿＿ 米

S3 级检测原始信息表-9　　　　　　　　　　　　　　　　文档号:＿＿＿＿＿＿

二次颗粒污染源	
二次颗粒源类型	☐机器 ☐工人
二次颗粒源位置	☐室内 ☐室外
与采样口距离	
二次工作模式	☐连续＿＿＿＿　　　　☐不规则间断 ☐经常间断＿＿＿　　　☐仅手动
备注	

参 考 文 献

[1] NNI. Environmental, health, and safety research strategy. National Science and Technology Council, Editor. Washington DC, 2011.

[2] Nalwa H S, Zhao Y L. Nanotoxicology. Stewenson Ranch (CA): American Scientific Publishers, 2007.

[3] Ge C, Meng L, Xu L, et al. Acute pulmonary and moderate cardiovascular responses of spontaneously hypertensive rats after exposure to single-wall carbon nanotubes. Nanotoxicology, 2012, 6(5): 526-542.

[4] Chen R, Zhang L, Ge C, et al. Subchronic toxicity and cardiovascular responses in spontaneously hypertensive rats after exposure to multiwalled carbon nanotubes by intratracheal instillation. Chemical Research in Toxicology, 2015, 28(3): 440-450.

[5] Zuin S, Pojana G, Marcomini A. Effect-Oriented Physicochemical Characterization of Nano-materials. //Monteiro-Riviere N A, Tran C L. Nanotoxicology: Characterization, Dosing, and Health Effects. New York: CRC Press, 2007:19-58.

[6] Powers K W, Brown S C, Krishna V B, et al. Characterization of the size, shape, and state of dispersion of nanoparticles for toxicological studies. Nanotoxicology, 2009, 1(1): 42-51.

[7] Borm P, Klaessig F C, Landry T D, et al. Research strategies for safety evaluation of nanomaterials. Part V: Role of dissolution in biological fate and effects of nanoscale particles. Toxicological Sciences, 2006, 90(1): 23-32.

[8] Teeguarden J G. Particokinetics *in vitro*: Dosimetry considerations for *in vitro* nanoparticle toxicity assessments. Toxicological Sciences: An Official Journal of the Society of Toxicology, 2007, 95(2): 300-312.

[9] Oberdörster G, Maynard A, Donaldson K, et al. Principles for characterizing the potential human health effects from exposure to nanomaterials: Elements of a screening strategy. Particle & Fibre Toxicology, 2005, 2(2): 8.

[10] Warheit D B. How meaningful are the results of nanotoxicity studies in the absence of adequate material characterization? Toxicological Sciences, 2008, 101(2): 183-185.

[11] Ge C C, Li Y, Yin J J, et al. The contributions of metal impurities and tube structure to the toxicity of carbon nanotube materials. NPG Asia Materials, 2012, 4.

[12] Meng L, Jiang A H, Chen R, et al. Inhibitory effects of multiwall carbon nanotubes with high iron impurity on viability and neuronal differentiation in cultured PC12 cells. Toxicology, 2013, 313(1): 49-58.

[13] OECD. List of Manufactured Nanomaterials and List of Endpoints for Phase One of The OECD Testing Programme, 2008.

[14] Dhawan A, Sharma V, Parmar D. Nanomaterials: A challenge for toxicologists. Nanotoxicology, 2009, 3(1): 1-9.

[15] Murdock R C, Braydich-Stolle L, Schrand A M, et al. Characterization of nanomaterial dispersion in solution prior to in vitro exposure using dynamic light scattering technique. Toxicological Sciences, 2008, 101(2): 239-253.

[16] Hackley V A, Ferraris C F. The Use of Nomenclature in Dispersion Science and Technology. U. National Institute of Standards, Editor. 2001.

[17] Shi J P, Harrison RM, Evans D. Comparison of ambient particle surface area measurement by epiphaniometer and SMPS/APS. Atmospheric Environment International, 2001, 35(35): 6193-6200.

[18] Ge C C, Lao F, Li W, et al. Quantitative analysis of metal impurities in carbon nanotubes: Efficacy of different pretreatment protocols for ICPMS spectroscopy. Analytical Chemistry, 2008, 80(24): 9426-9434.

[19] Sebba D S, Watson D A, Nolan J P. High throughput single nanoparticle spectroscopy. ACS Nano, 2009, 3(6): 1477-1484.

[20] Bello D, Wardle B L, Yamamoto N, et al. Exposure to nanoscale particles and fibers during machining of hybrid advanced composites containing carbon nanotubes. Journal of Nanoparticle Research, 2009, 11(1): 231-249.

[21] Powers K W, Brown S C, Krishna V B, et al. Research strategies for safety evaluation of nanomaterials. Part VI. Characterization of nanoscale particles for toxicological evaluation. Toxicological Sciences, 2006, 90(2): 296-303.

[22] Walton W H, Vincent J H. Aerosol instrumentation in occupational hygiene: An historical perspective. Aerosolence & Technology, 1998, 28(5): 417-438.

[23] Brook R D, Rajagopalan S, Pope C A, et al. Particulate matter air pollution and cardiovascular disease: An update to the scientific statement from the American Heart Association. Circulation, 2010, 121(21): 2331-2378.

[24] Balbus J M, Maynard A D, Colvin V L, et al. Meeting report: Hazard assessment for nanoparticles—Report from an interdisciplinary workshop. Environmental Health Perspectives, 2007, 115(11): 1654-1659.

[25] Maynard A D, Baron P A, Foley M, et al. Exposure to carbon nanotube material: aerosol release during the handling of unrefined single-walled carbon nanotube material. Journal of Toxicology and Environmental Health Part A, 2004, 67(1): 87-107.

[26] Methner M, Crawford C, Geraci C. Evaluation of the potential airborne release of carbon nanofibers during the preparation, grinding, and cutting of epoxy-based nanocomposite material. Journal of Occupational and Environmental Hygiene, 2012, 9(5): 308-318.

[27] Han J H, Lee E J, Lee J H, et al. Monitoring multiwalled carbon nanotube exposure in carbon nanotube research facility. Inhal Toxicol, 2008, 20(8): 741-749.

[28] Bello D, Hart A J, Ahn K, et al. Particle exposure levels during CVD growth and subsequent handling of vertically-aligned carbon nanotube films. Carbon, 2008, 46(6): 974-977.

[29] Fujitani Y, Kobayashi T, Arashidani K, et al. Measurement of the physical properties of

aerosols in a fullerene factory for inhalation exposure assessment. Journal of Occupational and Environmental Hygiene, 2008, 5(6): 380-309.

[30] Yeganeh B, Kull C M, Hull M S, et al. Characterization of airborne particles during production of carbonaceous nanomaterials. Environmental Science & Technology, 2008, 42(12): 4600-4606.

[31] Hsu L-Y, Chein H-M. Evaluation of nanoparticle emission for TiO₂ nanopowder coating materials. //Maynard A D, Pui D Y H. Nanotechnology and Occupational Health. Dordrecht, The Netherlands: Springer. 2007: 157-163.

[32] Demou E, Stark W J, Hellweg S. Particle emission and exposure during nanoparticle synthesis in research laboratories. Annals of Occupational Hygiene, 2009, 53 (8): 829-838.

[33] Peters T M, Elzey S, Johnson R, et al. Airborne monitoring to distinguish engineered nanomaterials from incidental particles for environmental health and safety. Journal of Occupational and Environmental Hygiene, 2008, 6(2): 73-81.

[34] Tsai M S, Fu W C, Wu W C, et al. Effect of the aluminum source on the formation of yttrium aluminum garnet (YAG) powder via solid state reaction. Journal of Alloys & Compounds, 2008, 455(1): 461-464.

[35] Piccinno F, Gottschalk F, Seeger S, et al. Industrial production quantities and uses of ten engineered nanomaterials in Europe and the world. Journal of Nanoparticle Research, 2012, 14(9): 1-11.

[36] Tsai S J, Huang R F, Ellenbecker M J. Airborne nanoparticle exposures while using constant-flow, constant-velocity, and air-curtain-isolated fume hoods. Annals of Occupational Hygiene, 2010, 54(1): 78-87.

[37] Methner M, Beaucham C, Crawford C, et al. Field application of the nanoparticle emission assessment technique (NEAT): Task-based air monitoring during the processing of engineered nanomaterials (ENM) at four facilities. Journal of Occupational and Environmental Hygiene, 2012, 9(9): 543-55.

[38] Methner M, Hodson L, Dames A, et al. Nanoparticle emission assessment technique (NEAT) for the identification and measurement of potential inhalation exposure to engineered nanomaterials—Part B: Results from 12 field studies. Journal of Occupational and Environmental Hygiene, 2010, 7(3): 163-176.

[39] Dahm M M, Evans D E, Schubauer-Berigan M K, et al. Occupational exposure assessment in carbon nanotube and nanofiber primary and secondary manufacturers. Annals of Occupational Hygiene, 2012, 56(5): 542-556.

[40] Dahm M M, Schubauer-Berigan M K, Evans D E, et al. Carbon nanotube and nanofiber exposure assessments: An analysis of 14 site visits. Annals of Occupational Hygiene, 2015, 59(6):705-723.

[41] Bello D, Wardle B L, Zhang J, et al. Characterization of exposures to nanoscale particles

and fibers during solid core drilling of hybrid carbon nanotube advanced composites. International Journal of Occupational and Environmental Health, 2010, 16(4): 434-450.

[42] Cena L G, Peters T M. Characterization and control of airborne particles emitted during production of epoxy/carbon nanotube nanocomposites. Journal of Occupational and Environmental Hygiene, 2011, 8(2): 86-92.

[43] Boffetta P, Soutar A, Weiderpass E, et al. Historical cohort study of workers employed in the titanium dioxide production industry in Europe. Results of mortality follow-up. Final report. Department of Medical Epidemiology, Karolinska Institutet, Stockholm, 2003.

[44] Sleeuwenhoek A. Summary of occupational exposure measurements associated with the production of titanium dioxide. Edinburgh, Institute of Occupational Medicine, 2005.

[45] Morfeld P, McCunney R J, Levy L, et al. Inappropriate exposure data and misleading calculations invalidate the estimates of health risk for airborne titanium dioxide and carbon black nanoparticle exposures in the workplace. Environmental Science and Pollution Research, 2012, 19(4): 1326-1327.

[46] Bałazy A, Toivola M, Adhikari A, et al. Do N95 respirators provide 95% protection level against airborne viruses, and how adequate are surgical masks? American Journal of Infection Control, 2006, 34(2): 51-57.

[47] Rengasamy S, King W P, Eimer C, et al. Filtration performance of NIOSH-approved N95 and P100 filtering facepiece respirators against 4 to 30 nanometer-size nanoparticles. Journal of Occupational and Environmental Hygiene, 2008, 5(9): 556-564.

[48] Kumar A P, Depan D, Tomer N S, et al. Nanoscale particles for polymer degradation and stabilization—Trends and future perspectives. Progress in Polymer Science, 2009, 34(6): 479-515.

[49] Mazzuckelli L F, Birch M E, Evans D E, et al. Identification and characterization of potential sources of worker exposure to carbon nanofibers during polymer composite laboratory operations. Journal of Occupational and Environmental Hygiene, 2007, 4(12): D125-D130.

[50] Methner M, Crawford C, Geraci C. Evaluation of the potential airborne release of carbon nanofibers during the preparation, grinding, and cutting of epoxy-based nanocomposite material. Journal of Occupational and Environmental Hygiene, 2012, 9(5): 308-318.

[51] Wohlleben W, Brill S, Meier M W, et al. On the lifecycle of nanocomposites: Comparing released fragments and their *in-vivo* hazards from three release mechanisms and four nanocomposites. Small, 2011, 7(16): 2384-2395.

[52] Sachse S, Silva F, Zhu H, et al. The effect of nanoclay on dust generation during drilling of PA6 nanocomposites. Journal of Nanomaterials, 2012, 2012: 26.

[53] Golanski L, Guiot A, Tardif F, et al. New method for the characterization of abrasion-induced nanoparticle release into air from nanomaterials. Proceedings of Nanotechnology, 2010.

[54] Wan Y, Kim D W, Park Y B, et al. Micro electro discharge machining of polymethyl-methacrylate (PMMA)/multi-walled carbon nanotube (MWCNT) nanocomposites. 2008,

17(4): 115-123.

[55] Wan Y, Kim D W, Jang J S, et al. Micro electro discharge machining of CNT-based nano-composite materials. //ASME 2007 International Mechanical Engineering Congress and Exposition. American Society of Mechanical Engineers, 2007.

[56] Cena L G, Peters T M. Characterization and control of airborne particles emitted during production of epoxy/carbon nanotube nanocomposites. Journal of Occupational and Environmental Hygiene, 2011, 8(2): 86-92.

[57] Schlagenhauf L, Chu B T, Buha J, et al. Release of carbon nanotubes from an epoxy-based nanocomposite during an abrasion process. Environmental Science & Technology, 2012, 46(13): 7366-7372.

[58] Wohlleben W, Meier M W, Vogel S, et al. Elastic CNT-polyurethane nanocomposite: Synthesis, performance and assessment of fragments released during use. Nanoscale, 2013, 5(1): 369-380.

[59] Van Broekhuizen P, van Broekhuizen F, Cornelissen R, et al. Use of nanomaterials in the European construction industry and some occupational health aspects thereof. Journal of Nanoparticle Research, 2011, 13(2): 447-462.

[60] Vorbau M, Hillemann L, Stintz M. Method for the characterization of the abrasion induced nanoparticle release into air from surface coatings. Journal of Aerosol Science, 2009, 40(3): 209-217.

[61] Gohler D, Stintz M, Hillemann L, et al. Characterization of nanoparticle release from surface coatings by the simulation of a sanding process. Annals of Occupational Hygiene, 2010, 54(6): 615-624.

[62] Koponen I K, Jensen K A, Schneider T. Comparison of dust released from sanding conventional and nanoparticle-doped wall and wood coatings. Journal of Exposure Science & Environmental Epidemiology, 2011, 21(4): 408-418.

[63] Jordan D. The adhesion of dust particles. British Journal of Applied Physics, 1954, 5(S3): S194.

[64] Kim I, Hwang K, Lee J. Removal of 10-nm contaminant particles from Si wafers using CO_2 bullet particles. Nanoscale Research Letters, 2012, 7(1): 1-7.

[65] Duncan R K, Chen X G, Bult J B, et al. Measurement of the critical aspect ratio and inter-facial shear strength in MWNT/polymer composites. Composites Science and Technology, 2010, 70(4): 599-605.

[66] Tsuda T, Ogasawara T, Deng F, et al. Direct measurements of interfacial shear strength of multi-walled carbon nanotube/PEEK composite using a nano-pullout method. Composites Science and Technology, 2011, 71(10): 1295-1300.

[67] Chen R, Shi X F, Bai R, et al. Airborne nanoparticle pollution in a wire electrical discharge machining workshop and potential health risks. Aerosol and Air Quality Research, 2015, 15(1): 284-294.

[68] Virwani K, Malshe A, Rajurkar K. Understanding dielectric breakdown and related tool wear characteristics in nanoscale electro-machining process. CIRP Annals-Manufacturing Technology, 2007, 56(1): 217-220.

[69] Meijer J, Dub K, Gillner A, et al. Laser machining by short and ultrashort pulses, state of the art and new opportunities in the age of the photons. CIRP Annals-Manufacturing Technology, 2002, 51(2): 531-550.

[70] Gattass R R, Mazur E. Femtosecond laser micromachining in transparent materials. Nature Photonics, 2008, 2(4): 219-225.

[71] Zhang Y, Gu H, Iijima S. Single-wall carbon nanotubes synthesized by laser ablation in a nitrogen atmosphere. Applied Physics Letters, 1998, 73(26): 3827-3829.

[72] Van Broekhuizen P, van Broekhuizen F, Cornelissen R, et al. Use of nanomaterials in the European construction industry and some occupational health aspects thereof. Journal of Nanoparticle Research, 2011, 13(2): 447-462.

[73] Koponen I K, Jensen K A, Schneider T. Sanding dust from nanoparticle-containing paints: Physical characterisation. Journal of Physics: Conference Series, 2009.

[74] Szymczak W, Menzel N, Keck L. Emission of ultrafine copper particles by universal motors controlled by phase angle modulation. Journal of Aerosol Science, 2007, 38(5): 520-531.

[75] Lioy P J, Wainman T, Zhang J, et al. Typical household vacuum cleaners: the collection efficiency and emissions characteristics for fine particles. Journal of the Air & Waste Management Association, 1999, 49(2): 200-206.

[76] Schutz J A, Morris H. Investigating the emissions of nanomaterials from composites and other solid articles during machining processes. CSIRO Nanotechnology Research Reports. March 18, 2013, Canberra ACT.

[77] Guiot A, Golanski L, Tardif F. Measurement of nanoparticle removal by abrasion. Journal of Physics: Conference Series(IOP Publishing), 2009.

[78] Zaghbani I, Songmene V, Khettabi R. Fine and ultrafine particle characterization and modeling in high-speed milling of 6061-T6 aluminum alloy. Journal of Materials Engineering and Performance, 2009, 18(1): 38-48.

[79] Ramulu M, Young P, Kao H. Drilling of graphite/bismaleimide composite material. Journal of Materials Engineering and Performance, 1999, 8(3): 330-338.

[80] Bello D, Wardle B L, Zhang J, et al. Characterization of exposures to nanoscale particles and fibers during solid core drilling of hybrid carbon nanotube advanced composites. International Journal of Occupational and Environmental Health, 2010, 16(4): 434-450.

[81] Pfefferkorn F E, Bello D, Haddad G, et al. Characterization of exposures to airborne nanoscale particles during friction stir welding of aluminum. Annals of occupational hygiene, 2010, 54(5): 486-503.

[82] Zhang B, Liua X, Brown C A, et al. Microgrinding of nanostructured material coatings.

CIRP Annals—Manufacturing Technology, 2002, 51(1): 251-254.

[83] Zimmer A T, Maynard A D. Investigation of the aerosols produced by a high-speed, hand-held grinder using various substrates. Annals of Occupational Hygiene, 2002, 46(8): 663-672.

[84] Park J, Kwak B K, Bae E, et al. Characterization of exposure to silver nanoparticles in a manufacturing facility. Journal of Nanoparticle Research, 2009, 11(7): 1705-1712.

[85] Li P, Xue W, Kim D W, et al. A Preliminary Study on Machinability of Polymethylmethacrylate (PMMA)/Multi-Walled Carbon Nanotube (MWCNT) Nanocomposites in Focused Ion Beam Micromachining. // ASME 2011 International Manufacturing Science and Engineering Conference. American Society of Mechanical Engineers, 2011.

[86] Koponen I K, Jensen K A, Schneider T. Comparison of dust released from sanding conventional and nanoparticle-doped wall and wood coatings. Journal of Exposure Science and Environmental Epidemiology, 2011, 21(4): 408-418.

[87] Khettabi R, Songmene V, Masounave J. Effects of speeds, materials, and tool rake angles on metallic particle emission during orthogonal cutting. Journal of Materials Engineering and Performance, 2010, 19(6): 767-775.

[88] Khettabi R, Songmene V, Masounave J. Effect of tool lead angle and chip formation mode on dust emission in dry cutting. Journal of Materials Processing Technology, 2007, 194 (1): 100-109.

[89] Zou B, Huang C Z, Song J P, et al. Cutting performance and wear mechanism of $Si_3 N_4$-based nanocomposite ceramic cutting tool in machining of cast iron. Machining Science and Technology, 2011, 15(2): 192-205.

[90] Ferreira J, Coppini N, Miranda G. Machining optimisation in carbon fibre reinforced composite materials. Journal of Materials Processing Technology, 1999, 92: 135-140.

[91] Nguyen T, Pellegrin B, Bernard C, et al. Fate of nanoparticles during life cycle of polymer nanocomposites. Journal of Physics: Conference Series, IOP Publishing, 2011.

[92] Göhler D, Stintz M, Hillemann L, et al. Characterization of nanoparticle release from surface coatings by the simulation of a sanding process. Annals of Occupational Hygiene, 2010, 54(6): 615-624.

[93] Tsuji J S, Maynard A D, Howard P C, et al. Research strategies for safety evaluation of nanomaterials, Part IV: Risk assessment of nanoparticles. Toxicological Sciences, 2006, 89(1): 42-50.

[94] Oberdorster G, Oberdorster E, Oberdorster J. Nanotoxicology: An emerging discipline evolving from studies of ultrafine particles. Environmental Health Perspectives, 2005, 113(7): 823-839.

[95] Kulinowski K, Lippy B. Training workers on risks of nanotechnology. National Institutes of Health, National Institute of Environmental Health Sciences, Bethesda, 2012: 43.

[96] Rouse J G, Yang J, Ryman-Rasmussen J P, et al. Effects of mechanical flexion on the

penetration of fullerene amino acid-derivatized peptide nanoparticles through skin. Nano Letters, 2007, 7(1): 155-160.

[97] Ryman-Rasmussen J P, Riviere J E, Monteiro-Riviere N A. Penetration of intact skin by quantum dots with diverse physicochemical properties. Toxicological Sciences, 2006, 91 (1): 159-165.

[98] Sayes C M, Fortner J D, Lyon D, et al. The differential cytotoxicity of water-soluble fullerenes. Nano Letters, 2004, 4(10): 1881-1887.

[99] Shvedova A, Castranova V, Kisin E R, et al. Exposure to carbon nanotube material: Assessment of nanotube cytotoxicity using human keratinocyte cells. Journal of Toxicology and Environmental Health Part A, 2003, 66(20): 1909-1926.

[100] Wang P, Nie X, Wang Y, et al. Multiwall carbon nanotubes mediate macrophage activation and promote pulmonary fibrosis through TGF-beta/smad signaling pathway. Small, 2013, 9(22): 3799-3811.

[101] Vankoningsloo S, Piret J P, Saout C, et al. Cytotoxicity of multi-walled carbon nanotubes in three skin cellular models: Effects of sonication, dispersive agents and corneous layer of reconstructed epidermis. Nanotoxicology, 2010, 4(1): 84-97.

[102] Murray A, Kisin E, Leonard S S, et al. Oxidative stress and inflammatory response in dermal toxicity of single-walled carbon nanotubes. Toxicology, 2009, 257(3): 161-171.

[103] Pauluhn J. Multi-walled carbon nanotubes (Baytubes®): Approach for derivation of occupational exposure limit. Regulatory Toxicology and Pharmacology, 2010, 57(1): 78-89.

[104] Golanski L, Guiot A, Tardif F. Experimental evaluation of individual protection devices against different types of nanoaerosols: Graphite, TiO_2, and Pt. Journal of Nanoparticle Research, 2010, 12(1): 83-89.

[105] Golanski L, Guiot A, Rouillon F, et al. Experimental evaluation of personal protection devices against graphite nanoaerosols: Fibrous filter media, masks, protective clothing, and gloves. Human & Experimental Toxicology, 2009, 28(6-7): 353-359.

[106] Gao P, Jaques P A, Hsiao T C, et al. Evaluation of nano-and submicron particle penetration through ten nonwoven fabrics using a wind-driven approach. Journal of Occupational and Environmental Hygiene, 2011, 8(1): 13-22.

[107] Golanski L, Guillot A, Tardif F. Are conventional protective devices such as fibrous filter media, respirator cartridges, protective clothing and gloves also efficient for nanoaerosols. European Strategy for Nanosafety, 2008: 1-8.

[108] Shaffer R E, Rengasamy S. Respiratory protection against airborne nanoparticles: A review. Journal of Nanoparticle Research, 2009, 11(7): 1661-1672.

[109] Rengasamy S, Eimer B C. Total inward leakage of nanoparticles through filtering facepiece respirators. Annals of Occupational Hygiene, 2011, 55(3): 253-263.

[110] BaŁazy A, Toivola M, Reponen T, et al. Manikin-based performance evaluation of N95 filtering-facepiece respirators challenged with nanoparticles. Annals of Occupational Hygiene, 2006, 50(3): 259-269.

[111] Rengasamy S, Eimer B C, Shaffer R E. Comparison of nanoparticle filtration performance of NIOSH-approved and CE-marked particulate filtering facepiece respirators. Annals of Occupational Hygiene, 2009, 53(2): 117-128.

[112] Kumagai S, Matsunaga I. Approaches for estimating the distribution of short-term exposure concentrations for different averaging time. Annals of Occupational Hygiene, 1994, 38(6): 815-825.

[113] Lee J H, Lee S B, Bae G N, et al. Exposure assessment of carbon nanotube manufacturing workplaces. Inhalation Toxicology, 2010, 22(5): 369-381.

[114] Birch M E, Ku B K, Evans D E, et al. Exposure and emissions monitoring during carbon nanofiber production—Part I: elemental carbon and iron-soot aerosols. Annals of Occupational Hygiene, 2011, 55(9): 1016-1036.

[115] Tsai S J, Hofmann M, Hallock M, et al. Characterization and evaluation of nanoparticle release during the synthesis of single-walled and multiwalled carbon nanotubes by chemical vapor deposition. Environmental Science and Technology, 2009, 43(15): 6017-6023.

[116] Fonseca A S, Viitanen A K, Koivisto A J, et al. Characterization of Exposure to Carbon Nanotubes in an Industrial Setting. Annals of Occupational Hygiene, 2015, 59 (5): 586-599.

[117] Lee J S, Choi Y C, Shin J H, et al. Health surveillance study of workers who manufacture multi-walled carbon nanotubes. Nanotoxicology, 2015, 9(6): 802-811.

[118] Hedmer M, Isaxon C, Nilsson P T, et al. Exposure and emission measurements during production, purification, and functionalization of arc-discharge-produced multi-walled carbon nanotubes. Annals of Occupational Hygiene, 2014, 58(3): 355-379.

[119] Tsai S J, Ada E, Isaacs J A, Ellenbecker M J. Airborne nanoparticle exposures associated with the manual handling of nanoalumina and nanosilver in fume hoods. Journal of Nanoparticle Research, 2009, 11: 147-161.

[120] Tsai S J, Hofman M, Hallock M, Ada E, Kong J, Ellenebecker M. Characterisation and evaluation of nanoparticle release during the synthesis of single-walled and multiwalled carbon nanotubes by chemical vapour deposition. Environmental Science and Technolgoy, 2009, 43: 6017-6023.

[121] Brouwer D, van Duuren-Stuurman B, Berges M, Jankowska E, Bard Delphine, Mark D. From workplace air measurement results toward estimates of exposure? Development of strategy to assess exposure to manufactured nano-objects. Journal of Nanoparticle Research, 2009, 11: 1867-1881.

[122] Möhlmann C, Welter J, Klenke M, Sander J. Workplace exposure at nanomaterial production processes. Journal of Physics: Conference Series, 2009, 170: 012004.

[123] Manodori L, Benedetti A. Nanoparticles monitoring in workplaces devoted to nanotechnologies. Journal of Physics: Conference Series, 2009, 170: 012001.

[124] Plitzko S. Workplace exposure to engineered nanoparticles. Inhalation toxicology, 2009, 21(S1): 25-29.

[125] Bae G N, Lee S B, Shin D C, Lee D J. Real-time monitoring of nanoparticles at a metal nanopowder manufacturing workplace. Proceedings of 10th IEEE International conference on Nanotechnology, 2010, 1183-1186.

[126] Wang Y F, Tsai P J, Chen C W, Chen D R, Hsu D J. Using a modified electrical aerosol detector to predict nanoparticle exposures to different regions of the respiratory tract for works in a carbon black manufacturing industry. Environmental Science and Technology, 2010, 44, 6767-6774.

[127] Evans D E, Ku B K, Birch M E, Dunn K H. Aerosol monitoring during carbon nanofiber production: mobile direct-reading sampling. Annals of Occupational Hygiene, 2010, 54(5): 514-531.

[128] Fleury D, Bomfim J A S, Vignes A, et al. Identification of the main exposure scenarios in the production of CNT-polymer nanocomposites by melt-moulding process. Journal of Cleaner Production, 2013, 53: 22-36.

[129] Ogura I, Sakurai H, Gamo M. Onsite aerosol measurements for various engineered nano-materials at industrial manufacturing plants. Journal of Physics: conference series, 2011, 304: 012004.

[130] Wang J, Asbach C, Fissan H, et al. How can nanobiotechnology oversight advanced science and industry: Examples from environmental, health, and safety studies of nanoparticles (nano-EHS). Journal of Nanoparticle Research, 2011, 13: 1373-1387.

[131] Tsai C J, Huang C Y, Chen S C, et al. Exposure assessment of nano-sized and respirable particles at different workplaces. Journal of Nanoparticle Research, 2011, 13: 4161-4172.

[132] Lee J H, Kwon M, Ji J H, et al. Exposure assessment of workplaces manufacturing nanosized TiO$_2$ and silver. Inhalation toxicology, 2011, 23(4): 226-236.

[133] Leppänen M, Lyyränen J, Järvelä M, et al. Exposure to CeO$_2$ nanoparticles during flame spray process. Nanotoxicology, 2012, 6(6): 643-651.

[134] R'mili B, Dutouquet C, Sirve J B, et al. Analysis of particle release using LIBS (laser-induced breakdown spectroscopy) and TEM (transmission electron microscopy) samplers when handling CNT (carbon nanotube) powders. Journal of Nanoparticle Research, 2011, 13: 563-577.

[135] van Broekhuizen P, van Broekhuizen F, Cornelissen R, Reijnders L. Workplace exposure to nanoparticles of provisional nanoreference values in times of uncertain risks. Journal of Nanoparticle Research, 2012, 14, 770.

[136] Wang J, Asbach C, Fissan H, et al. Emission measurement and safety assessment for the production process of silicon nanoparticles in a pilot-scale facility. Journal of Nanoparticle Research, 2012, 14: 759.

[137] Ham S, Yoon C, Lee E, et al. Task-based exposure assessment of nanoparticles in the workplace. Journal of Nanoparticle Research, 2012, 14(9): 1-17.